MW01034665

DATE DUE

WITHDRAWN

Cat. No. 23-221

Food for the Soul

Food for the Soul

Vegetarianism and Yoga Traditions

Steven J. Rosen, Editor

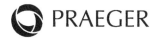 PRAEGER

AN IMPRINT OF ABC-CLIO, LLC
Santa Barbara, California • Denver, Colorado • Oxford, England

Library of Congress Cataloging-in-Publication Data

Food for the soul : vegetarianism and yoga traditions/Steven J. Rosen, editor.
  p. cm.
Includes bibliographical references and index.
ISBN 978–0–313–39703–5 (hardback : alk. paper) — ISBN 978–0–313–39704–2 (e-ISBN)
1. Vegetarianism. 2. Vegetarianism—Moral and ethical aspects. 3. Yoga—Psychological aspects. I. Rosen, Steven, 1955–
  [DNLM: 1. Diet, Vegetarian—psychology. 2. Food Habits—ethics. 3. Food Habits—psychology. 4. Spirituality. 5. Yoga—psychology. QT 235]
RM236.F66   2011
613.2′62—dc22   2011000975

ISBN: 978–0–313–39703–5
EISBN: 978–0–313–39704–2

15 14 13 12 11   1 2 3 4 5

This book is also available on the World Wide Web as an eBook.
Visit www.abc-clio.com for details.

Praeger
An Imprint of ABC-CLIO, LLC

ABC-CLIO, LLC
130 Cremona Drive, P.O. Box 1911
Santa Barbara, California 93116-1911

This book is printed on acid-free paper ∞

Manufactured in the United States of America

Contents

Introduction

Steven J. Rosen

Yoga and vegetarianism are popular subjects. Every year, more and more people are adhering to one or the other—or both. But these are also subjects that are often misunderstood, especially their interrelationship. Although Sharon Gannon and others have eloquently and convincingly explored this in several popular volumes, scholarly background and detailed references are much needed, representing a lacuna that the present book hopes to fill.

As I see it, my task in this Introduction is twofold: (1) to define Yoga, both in terms of its original meaning and in terms of how it is understood today; and (2) to define vegetarianism, so that readers become familiar with the issues at hand and how diet relates to Yoga.

To begin, the term *Yoga* is derived from the Sanskrit root *yuj*, meaning "union," "yoke," or "to join together."[1] As commonly understood in most Yoga circles today, this definition refers to a sense of harmony and balance between all aspects of creation, a connection to a oneness that engulfs all beings. This in itself speaks to the subject of our volume: How can one thoughtlessly consume the bodies of living entities with whom one feels kindred? How can one blithely exploit the creatures of the earth—who are a part of the same oneness as ourselves, who feel, and think, and enjoy—for one's own immediate pleasure?

But let us move on. Yogic union is also perceived as a sort of joining of the individual self with the higher self within, an awakening of spiritual consciousness, in which one realizes one's own divinity. This divinity is said to glisten with *sattva-guna*, or "the mode of goodness." Here, too, vegetarianism is implicit, for true goodness manifests in terms of compassion and love for all living beings. It's hard to love them if you eat them.

Ultimately, however, Yoga refers to a sense of "oneness in purpose" with the Supreme. It is, ironically, a dualistic philosophy of love of God, wherein one feels compelled to render devotional service, with a heart steeped in gratitude and affection for the Divine. Superficially, the "dualism" of Yogic perfection seems to run counter to the "oneness" mentioned above. The most evolved Yogis understand that the opposite of materialistic dualism is not monism, or total ontological oneness with the Supreme. Rather, the opposite of material dualism is *spiritual dualism*, wherein one gradually moves through a three-tiered hierarchy of spiritual realization, from (1) the materialistic perception that everything is separate and divided, to (2) a vision of spiritual oneness, in which one feels an intimate, loving bond with everyone and everything in creation; to (3) a higher spiritual duality, in which that conceptual oneness is bifurcated in such a way that *bhakti* (devotional love) can be experienced as the zenith of advanced Yoga practice.

This is an important step in one's spiritual development, for without this higher, transcendent conception of division—that is to say, without the "the making of one into two"—love cannot properly develop. After all, love is a phenomenon that exists between two beings, between one and another, not between one and oneself (except in the most narcissistic of material relationships). In higher Yogic awareness, one becomes established in the Self, realizing one's individual nature as a spirit-soul. This "spiritual individuality" reaches full maturity in one's loving relationship with God, a loving relation, in fact, that is viewed in the *Bhagavad Gita* (6.47) as the perfection of Yoga.

If, through Yoga practice or through other systems of spirituality, one is fortunate enough to realize the Oversoul of the Universe (*Ishvara*, as Patanjali puts it)—the source of all living and nonliving entities—not in theory but as a practical reality, one is then able to see the spiritual bonding of all things yet again. But this time it is a more mature vision, one that revels in simultaneous oneness *and* difference. As part of this advanced spiritual perception, "difference" now enhances oneness, so that the distinction serves the higher purpose of generating loving feelings toward all of creation, and especially toward God. Our interrelatedness is now understood as an eternal relationship under the universal Fatherhood/Motherhood of God, making us all cosmic siblings, as it were. We are all brothers and sisters through our common Father/Mother. Indeed, a Yogi who realizes this would never think of eating his more humbly endowed brothers and sisters, the animals, and this is the central theme of the book you now hold in your hands.

MENTAL MASTERY

Aside from this idea of union, the term Yoga is also identified with controlling the mind. Patanjai's *Yoga-sutra* (1.2), a seminal Yoga text, famously says, *Yogas chitta-vritti-nirodhah* ("Yoga controls the fluctuations of the mind"), leading to peace and tranquility. The original idea was this: Through the practices and methodologies of Yoga, one is able to calm the mind and gain mastery over the body. In this way, one can then use one's properly trained bodily vehicle for spiritual purposes—for meditation and for serving the Supreme (*Bhakti*-Yoga).

In the traditional Yoga system, this is accomplished through the *yamas* and *niyamas*, or the "dos" and "don'ts" of Indic spirituality. These are basically ethical rules and moral principles that lead to the proper practice of Yoga. According to Patanjali, the five *yamas* are

- Nonharming or nonaggression (*ahimsa*)
- Truthfulness
- Not stealing
- Refraining from sexual indulgence
- Absence of avarice

The five *niyamas* are

- Purity
- Contentment
- Austerity
- Self-study or study of spiritual scriptures
- Surrender to the Supreme Lord (Ishvara)

Many of the essays in this volume will look at *ahimsa* (nonaggression) and explain how this weighty concept impacts both Yoga practice and the mandate for vegetarianism.

One last note: Although there are many different forms of Yoga, the one most widely embraced by Western students is Hatha-Yoga, which centers around the physical body. This should not come as a surprise. The West is known for its attraction to the glitz of materialism, the lure of consumerism, and, now, the superficiality of New Age spirituality. This is nowhere as prevalent as in the modern-day Western Yoga community. Thus, outside India, the term "Yoga" is usually associated with Hatha-Yoga and its many variations and expansions, specifically its *asanas* (postures) and *pranayama* (breathing) techniques.

But the term Hatha-Yoga should be understood. Originally, the syllables *ha* and *tha* refer to the sun and the moon, respectively, pointing to the polar energies of the universe. The goal of Yoga is to balance these energies, resulting in consummate health and freedom from disease. Hatha-Yoga, in other words, is a system of physical maintenance that taps into the energies of celestial spheres, and it is thus especially meant for aspiring Yogis, because, as indicated previously, it helps them to avoid the distractions associated with the body, leaving them more time to pursue meditative techniques and spiritual matters.

Therefore, Hatha-Yoga is not merely a system of physical maintenance. Its methods function on subtle planes, directing the life force into all parts of the body—muscles, joints, glands, nerve fibers, and into each cell—allowing it to become a conscious and obedient instrument in pursuance of the divine. *Asana* and *pranayama*, it should be noted, are also said to stimulate endocrine activity, mediating the interaction of body and mind and aiding practitioners in the regulation and stabilization of thought and emotion. Thus, when properly adhered to, Hatha-Yoga nurtures not only the body but also one's mental and emotional responses to the material world, raising the consciousness in every way.

That being said, the more complete forms of Yoga, for example, Karma-Yoga (focusing on action), Jnana-Yoga (engaging mental activities and discrimination), and especially Bhakti-Yoga (the path of love and devotion), are considered "postgraduate studies" of the Yoga system, rendering imperfect all endeavors that do not move into these higher realms of spirituality. Indeed, Hatha-Yoga and its corollaries are meant to facilitate these higher disciplines, so that union with God might perchance actually become manifest.

Vegetarianism

"Vegetarianism" has become an umbrella term for a variety of diets that exclude meat, poultry, and fish. A "lacto-vegetarian," the most common strain of modern vegetarianism, refers to one who eats fruits, vegetables, nuts, grains, and so on, and also includes dairy products. A "lacto-ovo-vegetarian" consumes both dairy and eggs along with regular vegetarian fare—though here one is moving further away from vegetarianism proper. Some vegetarians, it is said, even eat fish, though most vegetarians would look askance at this. Finally, the most extreme of the vegetarian diets is called veganism, whose adherents only consume foods of plant origin, such as nuts, seeds, vegetables, fruits, grains, and legumes.

It is now well known that there are health benefits to a well-balanced vegetarian diet. According to the American Dietetic Association (ADA), vegetarians are at lower risk for developing heart disease; colorectal, ovarian, and breast cancers; diabetes; obesity; and hypertension (high blood pressure).[2] Overall, the vegetarian diet is considered a healthier option for humans in general, contributing to a superior quality of life. Thus, the desire for health and physical well-being that we see in the modern Yoga movement tends to overlap with the world of vegetarianism, which also offers a healthier lifestyle than the common meat-and-potatoes culture of the modern west.

But there is so much more. Another reason for vegetarianism is compassion toward fellow humans. It has been documented that the more meat we eat, the less we are able to feed the starving masses around the world. Global hunger, it is said, could be wiped out by adhering to a nonmeat diet. It works like this: If people worldwide took only 25 percent of their calories from animal products, 3.2 billion people would have food to eat. Not enough. Reducing that figure to 15 percent would mean that 4.2 billion people could be fed.[3] Much better. If the whole world became totally vegetarian, there would be more than enough food for everyone. The World Watch Institute sums it up as follows: "Meat consumption is an inefficient use of grain. . . . The grain is used more efficiently when consumed by humans. Continued growth in meat output is dependent on feeding grain to animals, creating competition for grain between affluent meat-eaters and the world's poor."[4]

And then there's the greenhouse effect and related environmental issues. *New Scientist* recently reported on the environmental impact of meat production, concluding, "A kilogram of beef is responsible for more greenhouse gas emissions and other pollution than driving for 3 hours while leaving all the lights on back home."[5] A letter written by the musician Paul McCartney and Dr. Rajendra Pachauri (who was a co-recipient of the Nobel Peace Prize for his work with the Intergovernmental Panel on Climate Change) sums it up nicely: "Vegetarianism is . . . a very attractive option for reducing emissions of greenhouse gases and stabilizing the Earth's climate, thereby ensuring global food security."[6]

Prominent publications—ones that do not generally cater to vegetarianism—have laid bare the negative environmental impact of meat consumption, lauding the concomitant benefits of switching to plant foods. In the April 9, 2007, issue of *Time*, for example, Bryan Walsh tells us, "If you switch to vegetarianism, you can shrink your carbon footprint by up to 1.5 tons of carbon dioxide a year, according to research by the University of Chicago. Trading a standard car for a hybrid cuts only about one ton—and isn't as tasty." Concurring, the March 2007 issue of *National Geographic* reports: "If, like most Americans, you get close to 30 percent of your calories from meat, dairy, and poultry, your diet contributes over 3,274 pounds (1,485.1 kilograms) [of carbon dioxide emitted annually]. Vegetarian diets contribute half that, but you can also replace your calories from red meat with fish, eggs, and poultry, for savings of over 950 pounds (430.9 kilograms)." In other words, a full vegetarian diet would be best, but a stepwise approach is at least a step in the right direction.

The above arguments for vegetarianism would appeal to those who are genuinely privy to the Yogic feeling of oneness with all beings, which mandates compassion toward our fellow humans. In other words, if one truly feels, or deeply understands, that we are all one, that we share this world as children of the same God, one never acts in such a way that would worsen our global situation, thus causing harm to fellow humans.

And what about the animals? They get the worst of it. Many vegetarians, in fact, abandon meat eating because of their concern for other species. Statistics confirm that at least 10 billion animals are slaughtered for human consumption each year.[7] This slaughtering takes place in "farms" that resemble Auschwitz or Treblinka.[8] These are not like the farms of our childhood, where animals roamed freely. Rather, most animals today are forced into "factory farms," where they are crowded into cages, without the necessary space to even turn around. Here they are fed a diet corrupted by pesticides and antibiotics. Tortured, they are finally released by a horrible death. Be it known: the law does not protect farm animals from cruelty, and so farmers, in general—especially those who eat meat— indeed treat them like mere machines. We exploit them for their "byproducts," like milk and eggs, and then cannibalize them for our main course.

Ahimsa

The entire meat industry runs counter to the Yogic principle of *ahimsa*, which means nonviolence or nonaggression. As we will see from the numerous essays in this volume, *ahimsa* includes not only other human beings within its scope, but animals, too.

Interestingly, the concept of nonviolence can only be expressed in the negative, by conjuring up the notion of its opposite—violence. There is no direct word for nonviolence in English or in most other languages. The same is true in Sanskrit, where the word for violence is *himsa*, and only by adding the prefix *a*—like adding the *non* to violence in English— do we get the word we are looking for, *ahimsa*. Thus, we only know nonviolence by what it isn't: it isn't violence. This speaks to the fact that nonviolence is simply alien to the usual state of affairs in the material world. Prominent thinkers such as Mahatma Gandhi recognized this and, based on earlier Vedic texts and Yoga traditions, fought for a deeper meaning of *ahimsa*, one in which it becomes greater than merely the opposite of *himsa*: in a deeper sense, it represents a higher love, total compassion, doing the right thing—qualities often found lacking in the material world.

The plain fact is that people in this world are steeped in violence, if not in gross forms then certainly in subtle ones. The world is set up in such a way as to engulf us in *karma*—an action/reaction schema that is forever binding. Even when we breathe, we kill thousands upon thousands of microorganisms. There is no escaping it, unless, of course, we use that same breath for divine purposes. Apropos of this, Yoga seeks to counterbalance material life's penchant for harm, first through *pranayama* and then through the chanting of Vedic *mantras*. When perfected in *bhakti*-Yoga, this leads to *hari-kirtan* (chanting the names of God), which manifests either when one uses his or her life-breath to chant the names of God directly or when hearing such chanting. An extended definition of *kirtan* (*sankirtan*) involves spreading divine wisdom and love through conversation, literature, art, and culture. All are forms of *kirtan*, the perfection of *ahimsa*.

ABOUT FOOD FOR THE SOUL

This book is a scholarly yet accessible treatment of vegetarianism in various Yoga traditions. It is a collection of authoritative essays both from the academic community and from the Yoga world. Hopefully, it will answer a pivotal question now being asked in books, magazine articles, and in everyday Yoga classes—just what is the place of compassion for animals and the vegetarian diet among practitioners of Yoga? Here, in fact, you will find a vast gamut of answers, drawing on history, philosophy, ancient Yoga texts, Hindu scriptures, comparative religion, contemporary practitioners, the words of sages, and the teachings of Yogic masters. This text elucidates the subject in a comprehensive and alluring style, allowing a variety of readers—whether students of Hinduism, practitioners of Yoga, vegetarian or animal rights advocates, or just people with a genuine interest—entrance into a provocative and edifying arena of philosophical speculation and understanding.

We open the book in an unlikely way: We question our central thesis and even give reasons for doubting its conclusions. Though the overall teaching of this book is that one must be vegetarian to properly practice Yoga, E. H. Rick Jarow explores dissenting voices in a diverse tradition, uncovering aspects of Yogic teaching that run counter to the vegetarian ideal. He allows previously unexplored nuances to unfold, perspectives that challenge the notion of Yogic vegetarianism. His paper also considers issues of cultural prejudice and idealistic and Orientalist projections by Westerners onto Indian Yogic traditions. I hope that this will lead to deep contemplation and the questioning of truths that have long been considered beyond question.

After Jarow plays devil's advocate, goading the reader to think deeply about the issues involved, my own essay more directly answers the question of whether one can legitimately practice Yoga and still eat meat. There are many possible ways to answer this question, of course, and this is Jarow's main point. Nonetheless, given certain overarching parameters, it becomes clear that vegetarianism has always been part of the Yogic tradition, and for good reason. Thus, my initial piece will set boundaries, define terms, and otherwise look at related issues in such a way as to more clearly explain why Yoga and vegetarianism are necessary bedfellows.

After this, the other, more detailed, essays in the volume will elaborate and explain things in their own way, according to the discipline or lineage they represent. Naturally, because our central theme—namely, vegetarianism and the Yogic tradition—permeates each essay, there will be a certain amount of overlap and repetition. Even this, however, has a positive dimension, serving to drive the point home more effectively and with greater emphasis.

As but one example of repetition that serves to emphasize an important point: Although I briefly examine *ahimsa* in my initial essay, *Edwin F. Bryant* goes into greater detail in his, analyzing Patanjali's original meaning of the word along with the perceptions and elaborations of other well-known commentators as they explicate the nature of the word as used pervasively in Yoga literature. Each of the essays in this book will examine *ahimsa* in its own way—to some degree, since it is a fundamental precept undergirding the entire Yogic landscape.

After this, we immediately start to look at the established Yoga lineages and what they say on the subject: *Kino MacGregor* takes us to the heart of *Ashtanga* Yoga, the Eightfold Path, confirming that Sri T. Krishnamacharya, Sri K. Pattabhi Jois, and B. K. S. Iyengar—veritable symbols of the modern Yoga tradition in their own right—espouse a vegetarian diet as being the best diet for spiritual development. This is a *sattvic*, or peaceful, diet, writes MacGregor, which prepares the practitioner's mind for the inner state of union and nonviolence that is the heart of Yoga. Here MacGregor offers an almost stream-of-consciousness essay that shows how one can gradually understand the importance of vegetarianism, and, more, how the reasons behind our diet are more important than what we do or do not eat.

And while we are sharing the views of established Yoga masters, *Rev. Kumari de Sachy* enlightens us with the views of Swami Satchidananda, her guru—using his books and numerous public talks as her source—in which a universal, nonsectarian approach to the subject unfolds. Here we learn how kindness to all creatures relates to mind, body, and spirit.

Natalie J. Ullmann, a long-time faculty member at the Jivamukti Yoga School in New York, draws on methods found in Patanjali's *Yoga-sutra* and on contemporary thinking in the realm of food and consciousness.

Her chapter explores the way in which meat eating opposes spiritual progress and the happiness and joy that is promised in the practice of Yoga.

David P. Carter and *Marguerite Regan* then show that Maharishi Mahesh Yogi, too, supported the vegetarian ideal.

After this, we step back in history a bit, as *Christopher Key Chapple* explores the hoary origins of *ahimsa*. His focus is the Jain tradition, an ancient Yogic path that views nonviolence as its central principle. The essay traces the "ensouledness" of all life forms, leading to vegetarian advocacy, especially as found in early Jain literature (*Acharanga Sutra*, ca. 300 BCE), medieval biological treatises, and modern Jain teachings. Aligned with the "many souls" teachings of Yoga and *Samkhya*, Jainism, according to Chapple, regards each life form (*jiva*) as worthy of protection, and this, of course, carries interesting implications for the subject at hand.

For the sake of being thorough, I include two final chapters on *Bhakti-Yoga*, the culmination of the Yogic system. As readers of the *Bhagavad Gita* will know, Yoga is more than just *Raja-Yoga*, popularized as *Ashtanga-Yoga* or *Hatha-Yoga*. There are numerous strands of the Yoga system, and, of these, the *Gita* is chiefly concerned with Karma-Yoga (the Yoga of action), *Jnana-Yoga* (the Yoga of knowledge), and *Bhakti-Yoga* (the Yoga of devotion). These paths have much to say about diet, specifically vegetarianism.

Joshua M. Greene, in fact, offers us an engaging piece about *Bhakti-Yoga* and how the nonmeat diet is most assuredly a part of that highly evolved spiritual vision. His musings on food and the devotional tradition of love for Krishna lead directly to my concluding essay, which further explores the same subject. Let's call it *Krishnarianism*—for it goes beyond mere abstinence and asks for positive spiritual consciousness while partaking of vegetarian foods, in which every meal becomes an offering to the Divine. Indeed, it is through the tongue—whether by eating such divinized foodstuffs or by chanting the names of God—that one truly unites with one's Maker, effecting what can confidently be called the perfection of Yoga.

NOTES

1. For this standard derivation of the word Yoga, see Gavin Flood, *An Introduction to Hinduism* (Cambridge, UK: Cambridge University Press, 1996), p. 94.

2. Brown University Health Education online: http://brown.edu/Student_Services/Health_Services/Health_Education/nutrition_&_eating_concerns/being_a_vegetarian.php.

3. Frank Hennesy, *Global Hunger in the Twenty-First Century* (New York: Banton Books, 2005), pp. 8–10.

4. See Earthoria online: http://www.earthoria.com/global-hunger-the-more-meat-we-eat-the-fewer-people-we-can-feed.html.

5. See http://www.newscientist.com/article/mg19526134.500.

6. See http://www.brighthub.com/environment/green-living/articles/18363.aspx.

7. See Bill Strauus, *Stats on Animals Slaughtered* (Los Angeles, California: Bantime Books, 2010).

8. For a graphic comparison see Charles Patterson, *Eternal Treblinka: Our Treatment of Animals and the Holocaust* (New York: Lantern Books, 2002).

1

The Yoga of Eating: Food Wars and Their Attendant Ideologies

E. H. Jarow

I think I could turn and live with animals, they are so placid and self-contained,
I stand and look at them long and long.
They do not sweat and whine about their condition,
They do not lie awake in the dark and weep for their sins,
They do not make me sick discussing their duty to God,
Not one is dissatisfied, not one is demented with the mania of owning things,
Not one kneels to another, nor to his kind that lived thousands of years ago,
Not one is respectable or unhappy over the whole earth.

Walt Whitman, *Leaves of Grass*

VIOLENCE, PURITY, AND PRAXIS

A friend and colleague of mine once went half way around the world to visit a renowned healer in Cyprus, honorifically known as *Daskalos*, or "teacher." My colleague was a strict vegetarian. I am not sure what he expected to receive from Daskalos, but on his plate in the kitchen were two sausages. Now, this was an ethical as well as proprietary challenge: does he break traditional laws of hospitality and refuse an offering from the holy man, or does he break his own law of spiritual purity and consume animal flesh? Observing my friend's hesitancy, Daskalos looked at him and said, "In your past lives, you wounded people with swords, now you wound people with words." My friend ate the sausages and never regretted it.

The following discussion is about food and Yoga, and more specifically it is about the issue of vegetarianism (or nonvegetarianism) in Yoga practice. I recognize that most practitioners of Yoga have been vegetarian and that the teachings of *ahimsa* tend to support a nonmeat diet. However, there are significant alternative voices in the Yoga tradition, and for the sake of being comprehensive and clear, I thought we should present them in addition to the usual perspectives on the subject.

Yoga has become a marketable phenomenon in the West. It may not rival the meatpacking industry, but it has taken its place as a full part of the contemporary wellness movement as well as having become a mainstay of current "secular spirituality." From this platform, Yoga teachers and practitioners create, or adhere to, myths of origin and transmission of Yoga in order to support or promote their particular perspectives, which often include specific ideas and ideals about what to eat, what not to eat, and why.

Without being clinically exhaustive, I think it can be helpful to put the "food issue" in some historical perspective. By doing so, one can see how Yoga has morphed and continues to morph, as both a practice and a sensibility, as it moves from one social milieu to another and takes on forms that speak to each culture's major concerns. Likewise, looking at historical flows of Yoga and diet can help us remember that such issues are cultural ones, that is, they involve much more than individual choices and proclivities: they reflect the purview, ethos, and fragmented forces of whole societies.

Food wars and their attendant ideologies, moreover, have always been with us. As cultural as they may be, they push us to personal edges that we did not know we had; for both what we eat and how we eat are as intimate and personal as they are culturally requisitioned and social. There is a deep, pulsating nexus of issues surrounding food and its consumption that spills over into areas in our lives that we do not immediately connect with the dinner table: class hierarchy, sexual politics, economic status, health, social memory, religion, and self-awareness come immediately to mind. Just as the anthropologist Sidney Mintz traced the history of sugar and how it played an integral role in colonial endeavors in his work, *Sweetness and Power*, one might begin to chalk out a related work titled something like "*Sweetness and Yoga*."[1]

Yoga, like sugar, has now been imported around the world, and while it has offered the sweet promise of wellbeing and even higher levels of bliss, it has also carried with it a lot of ideas, practices, and ideologies around food and its preparation and consumption. Since the Yoga that is known to contemporary societies arose in India and is still marketed as an Indian import, any discussion about the relationship between Yoga and food is best understood in terms of its origins in India. At the same time, however, one of the projects of contemporary Yoga has been to strip itself of its "cultural bag-gage." Therefore, it may also be appropriate to begin by looking at ways in which Yoga traditions have revisioned, assimilated, and transformed themselves and their food ideologies in relationship with the particular cultures that they now operate in. That being said, it would be useful to begin by looking back at classical India—the culture that gave us Yoga—and some of its major issues and proclivities around food consumption, especially the eating of animals.

In the Hindu world, issues of violence, purity, praxis, as well as esthetics and ultimate spiritual attainment, have been traditionally described and understood through a logic based on gustatory and consumptive meta-phors. No matter what your philosophical predilection, spiritual practice, or belief system, what you eat is a signifier of who you are, at least socially. This is an embodied phenomenon, far from Cartesian speculations. It is not simply that you are what you eat, but that you are the eating process itself; for consumption, as Robert Svoboda notes in his work on Ayurveda, entails the need to dominate another and make its *ahamkara*, "ego," part of one's own. It is, thereby, the primary instinct for the survival and main-tenance of a separate self. Prior to the will to power, is the will to live.[2] Hence, from very early on in India, issues of diet interwove with issues of philosophical doctrine.

The Upanishadic period (in and around 500 BCE) saw heterodox anti-Vedic and Brahmanical forces critiquing a hierarchically rigid and highly ritualized culture that, developing out of the nomadic Aryan groups mov-ing into the Gangetic basin, based its rites and economy around animal sacrifice. In the fashion of what anthropologists call "sanskritization"—the appropriation of the "other" into your own mythological framework—the Indian Brahmins, on through the Epic and Puranic periods (circa 200 BCE–1000 CE), declared Jain and Buddhist heterodox leaders like Rshabha and Siddartha Gautama (the historical Buddha) to be avatars of Vishnu, the all-pervading deity and preserver of the world. The Brahmins likewise assimilated the Buddhist and Jain ideal of *ahimsa*, "noninjury," and its attendant vegetarianism into their cosmology, even if there were strands of it in the parent faith from its inception. One sees this assimilation rather clearly in the *Yoga Sutras* of Patanjali, where a number of Buddhist ideas and structures are employed alongside classical Brahmanical ones.[3]

The dialectical structure around which the Vedic and subsequent Hindu cosmological system turned, however, was not one of violence ver-sus nonviolence but rather one of purity versus pollution, under which other classifying categories were subsumed. Violence was polluting to dif-fering degrees, but was not necessarily impure. A warrior who killed and then died in battle, for example, was lauded and assured of attaining heaven. Warriors were expected to eat meat, and the *Manu Samhita*, the quintessential law book of the Brahmins, also sanctions meat eating for priests in the appropriate ritual circumstances.[4] Moreover, the context in which sanctioned and unsanctioned food is discussed in Manu is quite broad, and seems to turn around ideas of who is or is not pure or impure, and to what degree, and under what circumstances. There are, of course, a number of well-known graphic polemics against meat eating in Manu:

> As many hairs as there are on the body of the sacrificial animal that he kills for no purpose here on earth, so many times will he himself suffer a violent death in birth after birth. (5.38)

> A man who does not behave like the flesh-eating ghouls and does not eat meat becomes dear to people and is not tortured by diseases. (5.50)

> The one who gives permission, the one who butchers, the one who slaughters, and the one who buys and sells, the one who prepares it, the one who serves it, and the one who eats it—they are killers. (5.50)

Ideologues who cite such verses, however, usually fail to cite counter verses in the same chapter:

> The eater who eats creatures with the breath of life who are to be eaten does nothing bad, even if he does it day after day, for the Ordainer himself created creatures with the breath of life, some to be eaten and some to be eaters. (5.30)

> Someone who eats meat, after honoring the gods and ancestors, when he has bought it or killed it himself, or has been given it by someone else, does nothing bad. (5.31)[5]

The *Manu Samhita* seems to be more concerned with context, therefore, than with essentialist ethics. This contextual characteristic of Indian thinking in general was well discussed by A. K. Ramanujan in his seminal essay, "Is There an Indian Way of Thinking," in which he remarks that from grammar, to esthetics, to linguistics, to dietary regimens, the classical Indian vision of appropriate conduct and action has generally been focused on particulars rather than universals. Manu, for example, gives a long list of animals that cannot be eaten (carnivorous birds, whole-hoofed animals, parrots, and fish, to name a few). Fish are said to be particularly impure because as scavengers they eat other animals; so someone who eats fish is "an eater of every animal's meat" (5.15). "Sheat-fish, red fish, striped and lion-faced, and scaly fish," however, may be eaten (5.16). The prohibitions extend beyond the animal world as well. Garlic, scallions, onions, and mushrooms may not be eaten by the twice born (5.3). Moreover, a

Brahmin should not eat food offered in sacrifice by a woman, by someone who does not know the Vedas by heart (4.205), or by those who are drunk, angry, or ill. He should neither eat the food of a thief, a singer, a carpenter, a usurer, a doctor, a hunter—and the list goes on. All these classes of people are considered to be impure and potentially polluting for the Brahmin.

As one looks further into this, one sees how the axis of consumption turns around the ritual purity of the Brahmins and their need to maintain their elevated status in society. Since context rules ethics here, Krishna can persuade the warrior Arjuna to fight in the Bharata war, despite Arjuna's abjuration of the ensuing bloodbath, for a warrior does well to fight, kill, and die in a just war. Likewise, the slaughtering of an animal according to the ritual prescription of the Brahmins was not thought to incur the negative karmic reactions that became associated with the eating of animal flesh by certain caste groups.

THE STRATEGY OF SACRIFICE

If there is one constant in the various strands of classical Indian ideas about food preparation and consumption, it is sacrifice. The offering of foodstuff to the gods and ancestors is crucial, central, and arguably more important than the objects of consumption themselves. In this sense, Indian tradition recognized the problem around violence and ego-domination early on in the Vedic period, well before both Manu and the Epics. I use the word "strategy" because it is a calculated response to the inevitable violence that any form of eating and consumption entail. As opposed to a strategy of renunciation, trying to get out of violence and consumption altogether, the strategy of sacrifice seeks to even out the playing field of slaughter by establishing rules of indebtedness. Hence, the ongoing centrality of *yajna*, usually translated as "sacrifice," but perhaps more clearly understood through the somewhat awkward nomenclature of "sacral transaction."

Understanding that violence is as inevitable as breathing, and taking off from dictums such as *jivo jivasya jivanam (Bhagavata Purana 1.13.47)* that "life lives upon life," the Vedic and subsequent classical Indian tradition established the practice of ritual offerings, reenacting cosmic processes of giving and receiving. Even the Supreme Person, *Purusha*, took part in this practice by allowing Himself to be sacrificed and dismembered, thus transforming into the phenomenal world. In this way, "equilibrium of exchange" is established. If you take, in the form of killing, you also give, in the form of offering the kill to the appropriate parties (gods, Brahmins, etc.), hence maintaining the turning of the cosmic wheel of ritual transaction.

The primary practice in the Vedic period was animal sacrifice: horses, cows, and other animals were prescribed as offerings for specific remunerations. The post-Vedic Brahmins did their best to minimize the obvious one-sidedness of this exchange (with the animals getting the worst of it), claiming for example that the sacrificed animal would immediately take another and better incarnation due to the efficacy of the Vedic mantras; and likewise was the claim issued that the practice of *yajna* was a step up from unbounded slaughter for gratification and appeasement of hunger alone. Indeed, it was a step up, for in sacrifice there is a recognition that some form of mutual exchange must exist between living beings, and that humans can become conscious participants in the cosmos through such forms of ritual exchange. The Upanishadic authors moved the concept of sacrifice further into the figurative realm, declaring the dawn to be the head of the sacrificial horse; the luminaries his eyes, and so on. Likewise, the fire of the altar and the heat it generated become internalized as Yogic heat, or *tapas*. Sacrifice came to be understood and discussed in many forms, such as making an offering of one's breathing, one's work, one's mind, and the like.[6]

This notion is articulated in the *Bhagavad-gita* when Krishna speaks of Yogic practitioners sacrificing their in-breath to their out-breath. With regard to food, the *Gita* is very clear about its sense of sacrifice when it declares that those who eat food offered in sacrifice are freed from all offenses, while those who are sinful, cook and eat food only for themselves (3.13). There is nothing discussed in these verses about what one should eat. How one should eat, however, is paramount. The *Gita* later goes on to list various foods that are situated along specific qualities of nature, furthering the notion of context, since those conditioned by specific *gunas*—qualities or "strands" of nature—will naturally prefer certain types of food.

Beyond this, however, is a greater notion of sacrifice: the *Gita* declares that since action (*karma*) is born of the Absolute (*Brahman*), it is eternally situated in sacrifice. Here, sacrifice is seen in its anagogical context. It is not just a question of particular substances being appropriate for particular people, but rather it is the notion that any and all action (*karma*) is incomplete without being linked to the whole. When linked to the whole, one understands that the food itself, the offering, and the one who offers are all *Brahman*. Yoga is this link. Hence, any action that is performed in this spirit is said to be Yoga. The *Gita* is clear on this when it declares Yoga to be "skill in action" (*yogah karmasu kaushalam*, 2.50).

This notion of Yoga in the *Bhagavad-gita* is all encompassing. But there is one verse in particular in which this "skill in action" is sometimes extended to the foods one should eat—at least according to certain modern commentators. This verse, it should be noted, focuses, once again, on the notion of context, or the attitude with which food is prepared and offered, more than with what one should or should not eat: *Patram push-pam phakam toyam yo me bhaktya prayacchati/tad aham bhakty-upahritam ashnami prayatātmanah*—"If one offers me a leaf, a flower, fruit, or water with *bhakti*, I will eat such things from this pure entity" (9. 26). Devotional commentators have used this verse as a sort of "proof" that one should not eat meat, since Krishna supposedly accepts only the listed offerings. The verse, of course, tells us nothing about offerings that are not accepted. Additionally, if one follows this logic, one could also eschew dairy products, sweets, or grains, since they are not mentioned in this verse, either.

What *is* mentioned, significantly, is *bhakti*, a word that can be understood as an inversion of, or better yet, the ultimate transformation of, mundane enjoyment. In the secular world, actions are carried out for the pleasure and aggrandizement of a separated ego-self, and generally not as a *yajna*. The Sanskrit word for "enjoyment," in fact, is the same as the word for "eating"—when that eating is enacted instinctively and habitually, in animal-like fashion. *Bhakti* marks the transformation from "eating" to "offering" and from mundane enjoyment to divine bliss.

This is all highly idealistic, of course, and ideals and living cultures are strange bedfellows. It is not at all uncommon for people to profess a particular position (*ahimsa*, for example) and then to go on to act in a completely contrary manner. Perhaps this is why the Great Epic (*Mahabharata*) continually reminds its audience that "dharma is subtle," as the ghastly Bharata war is referred to as a "great sacrifice." The genius of classical Indian culture, however, might very well have been its ability to accommodate any and all positions by making dharma not only subtle but contextual. As we shall see, emerging Indian religious culture was able to placate both vegetarians and carnivores.

The great theistic traditions of India began to emerge during the Epic period. In terms of their respective religious cultures, Vaishnava deities do not accept meat offerings while other deities, Shakta deities in particular, may. This is corroborated by the work of K. N. Sharma, who saw vegetarianism as even more aligned with Vaishnavism than with Brahmanism.[7] Some traditional texts try to negotiate between various vegetarian and nonvegetarian positions, such as the *Brahmavaivarta Purana*, which acknowledges that the sacrifice of animals gratifies the deity Durga, even while simultaneously subjecting one to the sin of destroying animal life.[8] In its spirit of "one *and* another" as opposed to "one *or* another," Shakta apologists explain that one who offers meat to the goddess transcends caste and ordinary rules along with all dualistic visions of morality.

While the medieval and postmedieval ascension of more nonviolent Vaishnava and Shaivate modes of worship and culture made vegetarianism

more popular, the trend was reversed through the rise of modern materialistic and secular culture. These perspectives, furthermore, become exceed-
ingly nuanced, because almost any behavior can be envisioned within the
purview of *svabhava karma*, "one's own righteous action," determined by
kala (time) and *sthana* (place), as the *shastras* (various scriptures) provide
for change required by circumstances. R. S. Khare, for example, discusses
the sanctioned meat eating of the Kanya-kubja Brahmins of the Katyayan
Gotra. This *gotra*, or lineage, harkens back to its ancestor, Vishvamitra,
warrior-turned-Brahmin, to validate its dietary regimen.

Khare finds that the Kanya-kubja Brahmins of higher education and
economic condition are more likely to eat meat, although it seems more
common in the Hindu tradition for people to become vegetarian in their
old age. This, interestingly enough, supports Carol Adams's contention,
developed through the study of European cultures, that meat eating has
functioned as a marker for masculine social power and success.[9] Indeed,
Khare notes that among these Brahmins, the consumption of animal flesh
is almost solely a masculine prerogative. This would all be quite compre-
hensible to Manu, who would see the *"rajasic"* pursuit of power and
wealth, the province of men, as corresponding to eating meat. Interestingly enough, in this regard, the Indian medical tradition, Ayurveda, has
no qualms about prescribing meat, and many kinds of meat, to sustain or
improve health and as a part of one's general diet in the cooler months
of the year.[10] Again, this makes sense within the *rajasic* realm, the hot
pursuit of the "good life" on earth, and indeed later commentators on
Ayurveda cast the meat-eating issue in terms of the conflicting interests
of health versus *dharma* ("duty," or "life purpose"). The Yoga tradition in
India, however, generally saw this from another perspective entirely.

THE YOGA TRADITIONS

Brahmanical notions about meat eating as being congruent with the
quest for wealth and power are significant and interesting, because contemporary Yoga traditions often align themselves more with the pursuit
of power and wealth (as well as good health and good sex) than with a
more traditional perspective of renunciation. Still, one should make no
mistake about it: the principal discourse of the Yoga tradition in India
has been one of renunciation. Yoga praxis has primarily been about *moksha*
("liberation"), focusing on freedom from the cycle of birth and death, and
in this sense it opposes the interests of both *dharma* and health-promoting
texts (as well as texts on statecraft and esthetics).

The word "Yoga," of course, has become ubiquitous, perhaps more so in
contemporary than classical culture. Although contemporary schools of

Yoga like to reify Patanjali as the "founder" of Yoga, Patanjali is clearly codifying an older, more diffuse, and largely oral tradition. Indeed the word "Yoga" is used some 36 times in the *Bhagavad-gita* in a variety of contexts and can thus be translated in many ways. The *Gita* attempts to weave the discourses of *moksha* and *dharma* together in its ecumenical effort, and in fact may be much more of a foundational text for Yoga in the West than Patanjali. Nevertheless, a look at Patanjali clearly places the Yoga tradition in the ascetic realm, no matter how people try to humanize it, because the *Sutras* are a discourse of renunciation, promoting dispassion and freedom from all cravings. The physical body itself is viewed as an encumbrance (1.19); indeed, the entire classical notion of Yoga is to "yoke the mind" away from the senses. Food, and eating in general, is therefore an impediment on the way to Yoga. One may be encouraged to eat "*sattvic* food" to have the strength and disposition to practice, but such a diet also serves the purpose of dispassion. By eating fresh but nonspicy, sweet, or oily food, it is believed that one is less likely to become ensnared by the lower strands of nature. Foods such as meat, fish, eggs, garlic, and onions are not considered to be in the *sattva-guna* and are therefore theoretically avoided by Yoga practitioners.

The *Yoga Sutras* go even further than this. They actually decry the will to live, seeing it as a "*klesha*," a force of corruption. The will to live may then be envisioned as the basic principle of consumption. One consumes in order to maintain oneself in the face of everything and everyone else. The *Yoga Sutra*'s sense of spirituality is clear in this regard. If it debunks the clinging to life itself as a *klesha* or obscuration of consciousness, then it must debunk eating (not just meat eating), which as mentioned may be the deepest symptom of clinging to life. In the hagiographies of the heterodox Jain tradition, the *tirthankaras*, the founders of the tradition, were said to have starved themselves to death. And Hindu tradition makes the first of Jain *tirthankaras*, Rshabha, an incarnation of Vishnu himself, endorsing this paradigmatic action. I say "paradigmatic" here because ordinary people are not supposed to starve themselves to death; they are rather to eat only food born of sacrifice. Yogis, however, who starve themselves to death at the end of their lives, are glorified, as Jonathan Parry describes in *Death in Banaras*. When death approaches, an advanced Yoga practitioner is to stop eating and focus on the life airs in the body so that the last breath may be offered as one's final sacrifice. Such a Yogi has conquered the illusory will to live.[11]

Thus, in an idealized state of *samadhi*, there would be no consumption at all. However, there might conceivably be a kind of reversed idealized consumption by adepts who eat, not because they are goaded by the will to live, but rather to bestow grace upon their disciples by "consuming" their karma. But this is another issue. On the Yogic path of renunciation, even to enjoy the taste of food is problematic (as described by Gandhi in his autobiography, for example). Hence the prohibition against *rajasic* foods and substances: it is not that such substances are evil, but that they do not contribute to the project of detaching oneself from the desire for more and more. To sum up: context continues to triumph over essentialism; there is no single law for Yogic eating, just as there is no single *dharma*.

Nevertheless, the predominant context of the Yoga tradition is to master the movements of desire and to leave the world behind. Ironically, however, the world is symbolized by food in the form of Annapurna, the Great Goddess who is, indeed, "full of food." How interesting in this regard, then, that the historical Buddha only achieves enlightenment after eating food offered by a woman! The mainstream Yoga tradition, however, continued to reject the sensual aspects of food, just as the Buddha's colleagues initially rejected him.

There are two wings of the Yoga tradition that have tried to do things differently, however: *bhakti* and *tantra*. *Bhakti* can be seen as an evolute of the sacrificial tradition, amplifying it to such a degree that the offering of oneself—often through the form of offering foodstuffs to the deity—comes to be considered the highest joy. In this way, *bhakti* circumvents the Yogic polemic of renunciation and decries the paths of *karma-kanda*, socially sanctioned worldly enjoyment, and *jnana-kanda*, the introspective path of knowledge, as "pots of poison."

Bhakti inverts the Yogic effort to detach from the mind and senses by positing Purushottama—God, the Supreme Being—as the fountainhead of the mind and senses, along with everything else. By acting to please the root of all existence, everything is put in its proper place, and there is nothing to renounce or control. Vaishnava *bhakti*, as mentioned, has tended toward vegetarianism, and, ironically, toward renunciation as well. Although all of the world can be used in the service of the Lord, the more devoted servants tend to ignore the world, absorbed as they are in the ecstasy of devotion.

The Shakta tradition, out of which *tantra* evolved, took another path. The Shaktas like to say that the Divine Mother, the fountainhead of all life, gives her devotees both *mukti*, "liberation," and *bhukti*, "worldly enjoyment." How could the all-merciful mother deny her children anything? Out of this is born the tantric ideal that the realization of nonduality obliterates mundane distinctions between pure and impure, violence and nonviolence, and that this is the ultimate freedom; not a freedom of license, but a freedom of insight. Creating a culture of *bhakti* requires a dedication to a particular form of the divine and a specific *sadhana*, or "spiritual practice," that a community can participate in. This entails a consensus of myths, images, and activities that constitute the sacred realm of devotion. *Tantra*, on the other hand, can more easily thrive in a secular community due to its interfacing of secular and sacred. It too requires a consensus regarding its set of myths, images, and practices, but there seems to be more fluidity and integrative potential in *Tantra* Yoga at the moment.

Both of these forms of Yoga have significantly impacted contemporary Yoga in the West, which continues to grow as Yoga itself becomes more nuanced and diverse.[12] Within this diversity, the pendulum has swung back toward the world, the Goddess, and the fullness of food. The legend of Annapurna may be instructive in this regard. Shiva was arguing with his consort Parvati over the subject of food. Shiva declared it to be *maya*, part of the world's illusory nature and unnecessary for what was essential: self-realization. Parvati took offense to this and left the world, taking all the food with her. The earth suffered in barrenness and thus Parvati returned to Varanasi to set up a kitchen and prepare a meal for Shiva. He then appeared before her with a begging bowl, saying, "Now I realize that the material world, like spirit, cannot be dismissed as mere illusion." Parvati took the form of Annapurna and fed Shiva with her own hands.[13]

YOGA IN THE WEST

In the contemporary Yoga communities of the West, caste stigma around eating certain kinds of food is absent. Hence ideologies and their attendant arguments on what to eat and what not to eat manifest in different forms. Macrobiotics envisions the spectrum of nutrition in terms of cosmic "*yin* and *yang*" energies without extraneous moral considerations. The raw food advocates decry not only animal products of any kind, but cooked food in any form.

The popular Yoga community, which seems to be largely concerned with personal wellbeing in terms of health and good looks, is divided here. There are ardent vegetarians like those of the Jivamukti Yoga Center, whose website rails against the killing of 25 billion animals a year worldwide and whose leaders have established numerous animal sanctuaries. There are the Los Angeles-based Yoga lifestyle communities, whose "vegetarianism" includes the consumption of chicken and fish, but not beef and pork. Then there are proponents of engaging in an intense Yoga session to be immediately followed by pasta, red wine, and chocolate—since Yoga is meant to heighten one's sensual awareness.[14] And the house remains divided.

One Yoga teacher who "came out" as a meat eater on *The Huffington Post* website spoke of the "rampant judgment" around food in the Yoga community, calling it "yogier than thou" and argued that "Since we do not live in the time of the founding fathers of Yoga, we do not know what they wanted us to eat."[15] The other side, of course, sees this as crass pseudo-Yoga, driven by ignorance, passion, and greed. The Jivamukti Yoga Center goes as far as to declare vegetarianism to be the most important first step in Yoga practice.

Interestingly enough, and this is what I would like to focus on, the driving notions of vegetarianism in New Age Western Yoga seem to also be about purity in a certain sense, just like the predecessor tradition. In these cases, however, purity is more often than not conceptualized in terms of one's physical body, in line with the Western (and, even more, American) focus on the individual. In some other cases, however, there has been an even newer twist: a vegetarian or vegan diet conceptualized in terms of aligning with a larger ecological, planetary awareness. Nevertheless, and interestingly, in both classical and contemporary Yoga cultures, the rationales for particular diets often follow "logics" of purity, and it is the ethos of these particular logics that I would like to further explore in order to frame the contemporary meat-eating issue in a more fundamental context.

The primary question here really is not whether one should eat meat or not. If Subash Chandra Bhose's work on plant sensation has any merit (and even if it does not, enough work has been done to convincingly demonstrate the conscious awareness of plants), plants may feel pain, in their own way, as animals do. Where, then, does one draw the line between sentient and insentient? This may be the heart of the matter when looking from a moral perspective, and in many ways it parallels the most sensitive and divided issue of abortion. What is life? Where does life begin? Is the killing of an animal akin to killing a human? What determines acceptable and unacceptable foods for humans?

Plant, animal, human: from a classical Indian context, all are embodiments of *atman*, consciousness, in equal measure, while each is covered by different qualities of nature. From the very outset, therefore, the Indian philosophical tradition sees the issue of consumption and violence through the larger frame of how to relate to the realities of embodiment. Are fetuses separate embodied humans? Are human embodiments fundamentally superior to those of animals, and are animals clearly demarcated from plants? Ironically, both classical and contemporary paradigms of Yoga may be all too similar in this regard, for they both participate in a patriarchal spirit of domination.

Traditional Yoga seeks to escape nature through the power of the will. Contemporary Yoga often seems to want to control nature and bend her to its will (as in "shaping your body"). There are differences as well, and I shall discuss them, but the theme of dominance remains. To be fair, there is another rationale that is given by Yoga-based vegetarians, the same rationale used by the heterodox Jain tradition and others, which is to do the least amount of harm possible. Most reasonable people accept the fact that in order to eat, one must dominate other life forms. So, the question then may be: what does it mean to participate in this as mindfully as possible? Is the effort to be of no harm based on compassion or horror at the way things tend to be in this world? Does Yoga offer a way through the jungle of the eater and the eaten, or does it look for a way out of it altogether?

The domination of nature and consumption of animal food has often been tied to social hierarchy, with upper classes employing violence as a means of demonstrating their superiority over others. Indeed, feminist criticism describes patriarchy as "the culture of dominance." Might it be possible that we are so enveloped in this culture and history that anything else seems ridiculous and unnatural?

The ascetic tradition, of which the Yogic tradition is a part, on the other hand, sees the need to eat as a source of embarrassment, for it is not a choice, not a volitional act, but a necessity that overpowers will and reason. Hence, domination is turned inward, "yoking" the body and the mind in the effort to overcome nature. Patriarchy leads to world domination, Yoga to self-domination. But in both cases there is an effort to wrest control from the natural world and perhaps significant discomfiture or even shame in finding oneself to be a part of it. Perhaps this is one reason why contemporary Yoga schools eschew the word "yoke" as a translation for Yoga—preferring the word "union"—and why the ecological argument is brought in. The ideal of "harmony" is much more palatable to the contemporary mind than "control," and there are other issues involved as well.

What happens, then, when the discourse of renunciation and control moves into the province of economic power, into the culture of individual freedom and domination of the other? There are a number of potentials here, and they have all had some play. On the one hand, Yoga can become part of a "counter culture," part of an ethos of sustainability that does not need machines. Yoga can also serve as a corrective to the betrayal of the body by the abstract "mind-only" cyborg-leaning culture as evinced by the French feminist critic Luce Irigaray's discovery of Yoga.

On the other hand, in other cases, and probably in most cases, Yoga is co-opted, and placed in a capitalist niche. Los Angeles has, for example, its Yoga stars, who bring in enormous amounts of cash, images of *asanas* are used to advertise products, and Yoga aligns itself with the cash-rich regimens of health and beauty. In order to do this, Yoga must find a way to integrate with the feverish consumptive mentality of contemporary culture. One way to do this is to package and sell Yoga, but what about its polemics of nonviolence, nonclinging to life, and nonparticipation in activities that will further bind one to the wheel of desire?

This is a tall order indeed, and this explains the unbelievable explosion of *"tantra"* in the postmodern arena. Millions of websites and YouTube videos promote *tantric* exercises, sensuality, vacations, and the like. More significantly for our purpose, *tantra* offers a way out of asceticism. If everything is nondual, then meat eating is just part of the cosmic weaving of the universe. Moreover, if it is consumed consciously, it allows deeper integration than the dualistic refusal of whatever may be morally unpalatable (no pun intended). Perhaps for similar reasons, Yogic monasticism has not taken off in the West, for deeply scarred by Christian canons, the West has had to shed its asceticism, and *tantra* offers a way to do that.[16]

On a more profound level, however, the *tantric* tradition raises what may perhaps be the most cogent spiritual critique against vegetarianism (I would argue that the "world as web" ecological tradition offers another). This critique is most succinctly summed up in one of the narratives of the 84 Buddhist *siddhas* found in Keith Dowman's *Masters of Mahamudra*.[17] The story goes that a royal prince-turned-Yogin was performing difficult *tantric sadhanas* when he encountered a wise female teacher who told him that although his psychic centers and energies were quite pure, there was a pea-sized obscuration of royal pride in his heart. She then placed some putrid food in his clay bowl and sent him away. The Yogin threw the slop in the gutter when he thought the teacher was not looking, but she had followed him and upbraided him, saying, "How can you attain Nirvana if you are still concerned about the purity of your food?"[18] The Yogin realized that he was still holding some things to be purer than others and went down to the Ganges and undertook a 12-year *sadhana* of eating the entrails of fish that fisherman had disemboweled. His intention, Dowman notes, was to transform fish guts into the nectar of pure awareness. The fisherwomen named him Luipa, "eater of fish guts."

In the *tantric* tradition, the guru is said to have super-knowledge that includes insight into the exact way in which the disciple is caught in attachment and illusion. Therefore, the guru can prescribe a specific practice that is perfect for that particular disciple. In the case of Luipa, eating the fish guts that even the fisherman had discarded was the way of conquering illusory notions of pure and impure. From such a *tantric* perspective there is no *sattva-guna* (balanced purity), or *tamo-guna* (ignorant darkness)—there is just the grace of the Goddess. Luipa lived on fish guts for eight years and attained realization and full freedom by imbibing the lowest of the low (fish as the flesh of a sentient being may be horrific for Brahmins, but fish guts are not even seen as being fit for dogs).

What *tantra* critiques, then, is the elevationist notion that tries to remove one from the world, even if that notion is guised in the cloak of wanting to do no harm. From a *tantric* perspective, being an ideological vegetarian is akin to an addiction. "I can only eat pure food, breathe pure cool air, drink pure water. Only such things will leave me whole and pure." But in order to attain this, one must leave out half of the world; one must refuse the sweltering streets and their people who cannot afford pure food and the like. From a *tantric* perspective the issue is not what one eats, but how one eats it. A *tantric* should be able to eat anything because he or she sees food as spirit. Any "ism," as good as it sounds, can serve as a mechanism of separation, by having one grossly or subtly think or believe that one is better or purer than another and hence enforcing the *ahamkara*, the notion that one is separate and different from everything and everyone. The ongoing hidden slaughter and packaging of billions of animals for consumption serves a similar "anti-tantric" purpose: it takes one away from the world, objectifies animals as things, and tries to sanitize the terrible reality of consumption.

It is also no wonder that Goddess Yoga should fill in a number of popular gaps here, for the Shakta tradition also critiqued the polemics of renunciation, saying that the Goddess offered both *mukti* and *bhukti*, liberation and enjoyment. How could the Goddess refuse her children the sensual delights of the world? What is important is to know where these things came from. Traditionally, Goddess-based religion has been a lot less squeamish about blood, birth, and death, eschewing an elevationist hope of transcending the world for a deep acceptance of the changing world as the body of the Goddess.

Yoga in a Secular Society

I heard a story recently about a New Age vegetarian who had been chronically ill and went to see a healer. The healer looked him deeply in the eyes and said, "You're starving." "Yes," the patient agreed, "I know I am emotionally disconnected." "No, no," said the healer. "You are starving for animal protein. Your body cannot live without it."

I know of many who have come back to meat eating because their bodies could not sustain a vegetarian diet, which brings up a legitimate question. Can Western bodies, whose ancestors lived on meat, and who live in the land of the bison, be sustained long-term by a vegetarian diet? Many say they can. The food wars flare up again and again, but this is not just a matter of proteins and carbohydrates, nor is it about someone's definition of *himsa* or *ahimsa*. This is about the wolf in you, the animal in you that needs blood satisfaction to survive and that understands its place in the natural world. What if the entire vegetarian ideal is a new chapter in the age-old patriarchal denial of the body, the earth, and the naked truth of embodiment? I have a colleague at Vassar who teaches a "food course" and once a year takes students to visit farms and to witness the slaughter of animals. Most young Americans, whatever their dietary propensities might be, have never seen an animal slaughtered. Many people these days, in fact, only see major farm animals on screens. A tremendous respect for the natural world can come out of this experience—of seeing what goes on at a slaughterhouse firsthand—a new understanding of *jivo jivasysa jivanam* as well as a new respect for the complexities of consumption in which we are all enmeshed.

The ghastliness with which William Blake looks at predatorship in the poem "The Tyger" ("Did he who made the lamb make thee?") reveals a sacred truth, sacred in its etymological sense of being "accursed." Perhaps being carnivorous is indicative of our fallen state, as opposed to the eternal world where the lion lays down with the lamb. This is the position of certain Christian communities who note that no meat was eaten before the fall.[19] Can one reach this ideal, however, by denying the realities of predatorship and embodiment, by swearing to do no harm and then being angry at anyone who disagrees with you? People who work on farms know about life and death. They know that to plough a field for vegetables and grains requires the killing of thousands of living beings, and that crops (as well as animals) ruthlessly compete with one another for territory and resources. The natural world features both an amazing web of cooperation and an amazing web of mutual destruction, vying for life. And we are all a part of this, even if we would prefer to not be.

No matter what our religious or secular proclivities may be, the question of the human place in nature remains an open one. Are we here to dominate the natural world? Are humans somehow superior and above nature, spirit beings or consciousnesses destined to transcend the "root and vegetable world," as William Blake called it? Holding oneself as the proud vegetarian apart, as a pure brahmanical and godly being, may be a result of this deeply inherited sense of spirit/matter dichotomy. It may also be another defense of the separate self, another way to refuse the animal within us. Here, Buddhist tradition, having released the idea of an *atman*, or pure consciousness beyond the phenomenal world, and moved toward a philosophy of interdependence, is a bit more forgiving of, or open to, the omnivorous diet than is the Hindu Yogi. Contemporary Buddhist discussions of this subject never fail to point out how the Dalai Lama eats meat under orders from his doctor, for example. In this vein, one can argue that idealistic textbook vegetarians never live with the animals as Whitman might have, never get close enough to the world to participate in it, but remain like Luipa caught in concepts of purity and impurity.

After all, to kill an animal and eat it is so sacred and terrifying that it breeds totemic religion. It demands awareness, humility, and a relationship with the beings who have sacrificed their lives for you. Every time you eat, it reinforces the truth of interdependency, violence, and the demands of the instinctual nature. Akin perhaps to turning toward Mecca and praying five times a day, eating turns us toward the central reality of our lives: consumption, transaction, power, and sacrifice. All this is of course a far cry from contemporary slaughterhouses and animal farming, which ignore the natural world and its cycles, which refuse to acknowledge the sacral mysteries of killing and eating others, and which assume the right of humans to dominate and inflict pain on other life forms.

The building of animal sanctuaries, however, smacks a bit of rescuing cats. It may be the showcase of a suburban neighborhood, but it does not make a dent in the city. It is much like creating communities where all farming is organic and where all the water is pure—only to find that radio-active dust is blowing over your land as much as everyone else's.

Still, it is a principled start. If the Yoga community is going to move in this direction, however, it will have to acknowledge itself as political. It will have to step into the fray, and run the risk of winding up like the Cathars, singing as they were burned (or in our era, completely co-opted by capitalism). This may be a much better fate, indeed, than living on a marginalized island of self-proclaimed purity as the world passes by.

If we take the Yoga tradition seriously, it will ultimately ask us to sacrifice an ego-based pursuit of health and wellness. That is unless a new paradigm emerges that links wellness to transcendence and redefines "renunciation." This is a most interesting possibility, but wellness cannot be limited to human wellness alone. Instead of seeing humans at the top of the world hierarchy, instead of seeing it as our job to save the animals and reengineer the world, one might ask the question in the spirit of sacrifice, "Who may eat us?"

Interestingly, classical Indian texts like the *Mahabharata* and the *Puranas* say that we are being eaten by time, and they ask if we can we go gracefully into that good night. Perhaps Jesus was being amazingly clear when he said that it is not what you put into but what comes out of your mouth that is significant. I have personally seen and heard many believers in Yogic vegetarianism arrogantly refuse to dialogue with—and, moreover, even speak disparagingly about—those who look at things differently (and I am sure that the reverse is likewise true). If the compassion of consumption does not extend to the compassion of relating with other humans on this earth, what good is it?

What our lives need are neither more-efficient slaughterhouses nor more self-righteous "Yogier than thous" telling us "the truth." Instead, may there be dialogue and respect around the immensity of this and like questions and a revisioning of the relationship between spirit and nature—hence this volume. Indeed, there may be nothing more essentially primal, profound, and necessary than consuming and sharing food. And if Yoga is ultimately about a union with the Absolute, whether through love, knowledge, or *tantric* nondual awareness, can one's practice of consumption then move one toward such a union with generosity and open-heartedness?

NOTES

1. Mintz, Sidney. *Sweetness and Power: The Place of Sugar in Modern History.* New York: Viking, 1985.

2. Svoboda, Robert. *Prakriti: Your Ayurvedic Constitution.* Twin Lakes, WI: Lotus Press, 1989).

3. Patanjali's eight limbs of Yoga, for example, clearly resonate with the eightfold path in the Pali Canon as do the *yamas* and *niyamas*. Likewise, Patanjali brings in the orthodox and brahmanical tradition by invoking surrender to the Lord Ishwara as part of the prerequisites for Yoga practice.

4. Doniger Wendy, Smith, Bian K, trans., *The Laws of Manu,* New York: Penguin, 1991, p. 102. The *Manu Samhitia,* also known as the *Manavadharmashastra* and *Manusmriti,* was most likely compiled during the Epic period (200 BCE–200 CE) and deals extensively with the obligations of the four *varnas,* or social classes.

5. Ibid.

6. "Aum, the dawn, verily, is the head of the sacrificial horse, the sun the eye, the wind the breath, the open mouth the Vaishvanara [universally worshipped] fire; the year is the body of the sacrificial horse, the sky is the back, the atmosphere is the belly, the earth the hoof [or, the earth is his footing], the quarters the sides, the intermediate quarters the ribs, the seasons the limbs, the months and the half-months the joints, days and nights the feet, the stars the bones, the clouds the flesh; the food in the stomach is the sand, the rivers are the blood-vessels, the liver and the lungs are the mountains, the herbs and the trees are the hair. The rising (sun) is the forepart, the setting (sun) the hind part, when he yawns then it lightens, when he shakes himself, it thunders, when he urinates then it rains." *Brihadaranyaka Upanishad* 1.1

7. Sharma, K. N., "Hindu Sects and Food Patterns in North India," in *Aspects of Religion in Indian Society,* ed. L. P. Vidyarthi. Meerut, 1961, p. 53.

8. Ibid., p. 233.

9. Adams, Carol J. *The Sexual Politics of Meat: A Feminist-Vegetarian Critical Theory.* New York: Continuum, 1990.

10. See Dominik Wujastyk's discussion of this in his *Roots of Ayurveda: Selections from the Ayurvedic Classics.* New Delhi: Penguin Books, 1998. The seminal Ayurvedic texts of Caraka and Sushruta take meat eating for granted. It is only later commentators who raise the question of violence (such as Cakrapanidatta).

11. Parry, Jonathan, P. *Death in Banaras.* Cambridge, New York: Cambridge University Press, 1994.

12. On a recent Google search, there were 3,580,000 sites listed for *bhakti* and 6,750,000 sites listed for *tantra*. Yoga, however, largely outdistanced them with 67,600,000 sites listed.

13. Saraswati, Swami Satyananda. *Annapurna Puja and Sahasranam* (ISBN 18-8748285-1).

14. Moskin, Julia. "When Chocolate and Chakras Collide," *New York Times*, Jan. 26, 2010.

15. Ibid., p. 2, The Yoga teacher, Sadie Nardini, is quoted by Julia Moskin in the *Times*: "Nowhere is it written that only vegetarians can do Yoga."

16. For an extended discussion on this, see Hugh Urban's *Tantra: Sex, Secrecy, Politics, and Power in the Study of Religions*. Berkeley: University of California Press, 2003.

17. Dowman, Keith, masters of Mahamudra: *Songs and Histories of the Eighty-Four Buddhist Siddhas*. New York: State University of New York Press, 1985. SUNY Series in Buddhist Studies, ed. Kenneth. K. Inada.

18. Ibid., p. 33.

19. On the other hand, vegetarian Christians note in the same vein that just as blood sacrifices began after the fall they end with Jesus, who as the redeemer is the last blood sacrifice.

2

❧

Burgers or Buns: A Brief Look at Whether a Yogi Should Be a Vegetarian

Steven J. Rosen

"Oh, yes, I practice Yoga," she said, with great confidence. "I've been doing it—big time—for over 15 years. Making great progress."

"Are you a vegetarian?"

"Nope. Don't have to be. That's the beauty of Yoga—as long as you do your *pranayama* (breathing exercises) and your *asanas* (postures), you're okay."

It was then that I made up my mind: I needed to look into this—big time, as she says—once and for all. Could a person, in fact, be a Yogi or a Yogini and still scarf down an animal? Is it possible to practice *pranayama* and *asana* properly, in the sanctity of a Yoga studio, and then walk over to a restaurant or supermarket and unconsciously support the killing of our four-footed, feathered, and scaly kin?

Fact is, according to a recent survey on the website The Yoga Site: The Online Yoga Resource Center, nearly two-thirds of modern Yoga practitioners in the Western world are not vegetarians.[1] That's a lot of people. According to *Yoga Journal's* 2008 study, 16.9 percent of U.S. adults, or 15.8 million people, practice Yoga.[2] And there are millions more doing it elsewhere on the planet. In other words, tens of millions adopt a Yogic lifestyle without becoming vegetarian. Is that legitimate?

Many prominent Yoga teachers seem to think so, openly endorsing a meat-centered diet. Historically, to be sure, Tantrics and various kinds of Buddhist Yogis have included meat as part of their dietary regimen, and perhaps carnivorous practitioners today can trace the practice to these early Yogic traditions.[3] But the Yoga tradition, by and large, has eschewed the use of flesh-foods, largely on the basis of a nonviolent ethic, eating habits that favorably contribute to a healthy lifestyle, and a sense of compassion for all living things.

NOT BLOODY LIKELY!

That any Yoga teachers would encourage meat eating is interesting, especially if you consider the following: Though there are certainly exceptions, most Yoga lineages today can be traced to two particular stalwarts in the tradition: Sri Krishnamacharya (1888–1989) and Swami Sivananda (1887–1963).[4] Krishnamacharya brought forth teachers such as K. Pattabhi Jois, T. K. V. Desikachar, and B. K. S. Iyengar, whose practices manifest in the modern world as Ashtanga-Vinyasa, Viniyoga, and the Iyengar method, respectively. Sivananda, for his part, is represented today by the Integral Yoga Institute, Swami Satchidananda, Swami Chinmayananda, and so on. Thus, most Yoga practitioners today use the methods formulated by or inherited from these two men, either as they were originally espoused or in conjunction with other methods.

Here is the interesting part: Krishnamacharya descends from the Shri Vaishnava lineage, which staunchly upholds the vegetarian ideal. We learn from his followers that he believed one could not properly practice Yoga without giving up meat.[5] And Sivananda, too, was an outspoken vegetarian. For proof, one need look no further than his popular essay, "Swami Sivananda on Vegetarian Diet."[6] Given this meat-free background, one might understandably utter the mantra: "What gives? Why do numerous Yoga institutions and teachers lean toward meat eating?"

To be fair, there are Yoga teachers who have championed the vegetarian ideal, even if they are few and far between. The Integral Yoga people, beginning with Swami Satchidananda himself,[7] and Jivamukti Yoga immediately come to mind. Sharon Gannon, co-founder of Jivamukti, even published a seminal book on the subject, *Yoga and Vegetarianism* (Mandala, 2008), in which she lays bare the philosophical underpinnings of a nonmeat diet, both in general and in the Yoga tradition.

In the book, Gannon tells a story wherein Pattabhi Jois, one of her accomplished teachers, mentioned above, declares that vegetarianism is unavoidable for one who wants to be a Yogi. Writes Gannon:

> He was initially very reluctant to teach Western students because they were meat eaters. It was only in the last twenty years or so that he opened his doors wide to Western students. I had assumed the reason was that he felt there would be language difficulties, but when I asked him if that was why he refused Western students for many years, he replied: "No. It was because they weren't vegetarians. If someone is not a vegetarian, they won't be able to learn yoga."[8]

Jois is one of the modern era's leading experts on Yoga. So is B. K. S. Iyengar, also mentioned above. In his book, *Light on Yoga*, he is equally firm: "A vegetarian diet is a necessity for the practice of Yoga."[9] At times, Iyengar seems to hedge, but it quickly becomes clear what his beliefs actually are:

> Whether or not to be a vegetarian is a purely personal matter, as each person is influenced by the tradition and habits of the country in which he was born and bred. But, in course of time, the practitioner of yoga has to adopt a vegetarian diet, in order to attain one-pointed attention and spiritual evolution.[10]

In the light of this, meat eaters who call themselves Yogis would probably do well to ask themselves the following question: "Who are we to argue with Satchidananda, Gannon, Jois, and Iyengar?"

Of course, these four luminaries, among others, would not deny that someone could begin their practice of Yoga while still eating meat, especially if their intent is to gradually give it up. Indeed, fledgling Yogis come to the practice with all kinds of baggage, meat eating being only one amongst many. But serious practitioners should know well the importance of gradually leaving bad habits aside, including the eating of animals. Those who are intent on giving up deleterious practices are those who will make progress on the Yogic path.

To begin, then, it seems necessary to define what "practicing Yoga" actually means. There are certainly "part-time Yogis," if you will—people who attend occasional Yoga classes, or who use various techniques borrowed from the ancient system to get a good work-out, for the purpose of rounding out an exercise regimen. If you're merely using Yoga to acquire tight buns, it matters little if you garnish those buns with hamburger. (Of course, this is also open to discussion, since obesity and related diseases are much more common in the nonveggie world.)

But anyone claiming to "actually" practice Yoga, who does it to achieve the system's stated goals—bliss, enlightenment, conquering the fluctuations of the mind, liberation, union with God or developing love for Him—should indeed think twice. Research into early Yogic texts tends to show that it is simply delusional to think that one can actually practice Yoga if one eats meat. Indeed, making real progress on the Yogic path while eating meat is, to quote a famous Yogi, "just plain bull."

WHAT DO THE ORIGINAL TEXTS SAY?

The mandate for Yogis to be vegetarian comes from the larger tradition as a whole. Aside from countless verses that support this view in the Vedic literature, the Epics,[11] the Puranas, and the *Manu-samhita*, the truth of vegetarianism is based on Patanjali's original text itself. In his *Yoga Sutras*, which lay out the basis of all Yoga practice, he presents an eight-step outline for attaining liberation from material existence. The first step is called *yama*, which means "restraints." Here we find five ethical guidelines that must be followed by all aspiring Yogis: nonviolence (*ahimsa*), truthfulness (*satya*), refraining from stealing (*asteya*), sexual self-control (*brahmacharya*), and refraining from unnecessary acquisition, or greediness (*aparigraha*).

The very first of these restraints is *ahimsa*, which is usually translated as "nonviolence" but is also defined as "nonaggression" or "nonharming." The word's broad implications involve not only "doing no harm to any living being"—and the traditional Yoga commentaries make it clear that this also includes animals—but also, more positively, to be loving and to make the world a better place. According to Patanjali (2.30), this principle is the very heart of Yogic sensibility. That's why he places it first, before all other precepts. Not only that, but, in traditional Sanskrit literature, introductory statements tend to carry more weight than the rest of the text, often forming the basis for all that follows. Accordingly, the initial commentators on the *Yoga-sutras*, including Vyasa, the *sutras'* preeminent commentator, say that *ahimsa* is the root of all other Yogic instructions, which are properly practiced only when one understands and incorporates the principle of nonviolence.[12]

Gannon explains this clearly in her book by showing how *ahimsa* impacts the other *yamas:* For example, she says that *satya*, or "truthfulness," is compromised by meat eating, especially in the modern West. Most people purchase their meat nicely wrapped in supermarkets. "We don't want to get our hands dirty so we hire a hit man to do the murder and then pretend the murder didn't happen," writes Gannon. "It's not truthful."[13] She asks us, too, to consider the principle of *asteya*, or "not stealing": "All the rights we hold dear as humans we deprive of animals," she notes. "[W]e steal their babies, eggs and their lives."[14] If you are violent, you steal away others' sense of safety—this is true even if they're "only" animals. In this way, she builds a case, based on logic, common sense, and on the traditional commentators, that *ahimsa* must be followed by all who claim to be Yogis, and also that the following of all other Yogic principles is dependent on fully embracing *ahimsa*.

For those trained in Western traditions, *ahimsa* is reminiscent of the Latin phrase, *primum non nocere*: "First, do no harm." This is, of course, the basis of the Hippocratic Oath, a principle that all physicians and healthcare professionals consider primary in their treatment of others. This same principle should be considered in relation to the slaughterhouses and related industries that give us meat eating, which are violent from beginning to end. It is now common knowledge how factory-farms treat cows, chickens, pigs, and other animals, forcing them to imbibe unnecessary, harmful drugs, debeaking the birds, and otherwise subjecting them to horrendous living conditions. The cruelty inflicted on farm animals is inconceivable. Older, more traditional farms are not much better. The plain fact is that such places—even the best of them—are a violation of *ahimsa*, which cannot be tolerated by those who know the progressive values of life.

Edwin F. Bryant, professor of Hindu Religion and Philosophy at Rutgers University, concurs. His recently released translation and commentary on Patanjali's *sutras*—a massive repository of Yogic learning—rightly positions Bryant as one of the foremost intellectual authorities in the field. And after purveying the vast literature on Yoga, both by traditional commentators and by modern authorities, his words are conclusive:

> A sattvic [bright, conscious] person is empathetic and compassionate toward other embodied beings and would never countenance inflicting violence upon them, what to speak of eating their flesh. Moreover, being insightful, such a person understands the karmic consequence of violent actions. . . . Any involvement in violent acts of any kind requires that the perpetrator be subjected to the same violence at some future time as karmic consequence. Moreover, inflicting violence is a quality of tamas [ignorance], and thus eating meat increases the tamasic potential of the citta [mind, consciousness], further enhancing ignorance. A vegetarian diet is nonnegotiable for yogis.[15]

In other words, one who is cultivating higher consciousness will naturally be compassionate toward all creatures, which necessarily includes refraining from eating their flesh. In addition, Bryant points out, the karmic reaction of eating a living creature's flesh is that one must come back, in a future birth, to suffer a similar fate—this karmic consequence is validated in all traditional literature on Yoga and related subjects. Finally, Bryant mentions that since meat eating is essentially an act of ignorance, it perpetuates the ignorance currently found in one's consciousness, deepening it and establishing it as an irrevocable fact.

Other Yogic writings say much the same. For example, the *Hatha Yoga Pradipika* of Svatmarama (1.59), the most important Hatha-Yoga text after Patanjali's *sutras*, recommends avoiding "fish, meat . . ." and certain other foods, describing them as "not being salutary."

And the *Bhagavad Gita*, valuable in that it was originally spoken by Lord Krishna (also known as Yogeshvara, "the master of mystic Yoga") and because it teaches Bhakti-yoga, the Yoga of devotion—which is the culmination of all forms of spiritual practice—augments the *ahimsa* argument with its explanation of the three modes of material nature—goodness, passion, and ignorance—and how these qualities impact the food we eat. It tells us that *sattvic* foods (fruit, vegetables, grains, etc.) "promote vitality, health, pleasure, strength, and long life." Bitter, salty, and sour foods (including meat, fish, and alcohol), on the other hand, are rajasic, "causing pain, disease, and discomfort." And then there are foods in the *tamasic* category: "stale, overcooked, and contaminated," including rotten or impure foods.[16] Implicitly, a vegetarian diet is preferred, for who would not want the fruits of *sattvic* eating habits, or, put another way, who would want to suffer the consequences of a diet steeped in passion and ignorance?

From Vegetarianism to Divine Edibles

Yogis who are serious about what they eat will not only try to eat *sattvic* foods, avoiding those in *rajas* and *tamas*—especially meat—but they also try to fully spiritualize the experience of eating. "Food, the supporting yet consuming substance of all life," writes Iyengar, "is regarded as a phase of Brahman [the supreme spirit]. It should be eaten with the feeling that with each morsel one can gain strength to serve the Lord."[17] This is the mood of the true Yogi, who sees food as a manifestation of Brahman—nondifferent from God Himself—because it is offered to Him/Her with love and devotion, not only externally as a sacrifice, with *mantras* and rituals, but also internally, with a prayer that basically says this: "Whatever strength I gain from eating this food should be used in Your divine service throughout my life." This principle of offering food to God—and the foodstuffs that result from such an offering—is called *prasadam* ("the Lord's mercy"), and it facilitates Yogic perfection.

But *prasadam* must be vegetarian, and so one should clearly understand the value of a nonmeat diet. In fact, there are numerous, well-documented reasons for turning to vegetarianism—and each of these is good not only for the individual (and for the animals) but also for the world. Here is a brief summary:

- Believe it or not, eating animals contributes to global warming. A specialist report by the University of Chicago in 2006 found that a vegan diet does more in the fight against global warming than switching to a hybrid car.
- It takes up to 16 pounds of grain to produce just 1 pound of animal flesh. The inefficient conversion ratio in feeding plant foods to farm animals—whose flesh we eat—is not viable. It is more efficient to eat the plant foods ourselves.
- In the United States, chickens, turkeys, pigs, and cows in factory farms produce nearly 90,000 pounds of excrement every few seconds. This excrement is contaminated with the antibiotics and hormones that are pumped into

their bodies to increase their value as flesh meat. Thus, the U.S. Environmental Protection Agency tells us, the runoff from factory farms pollutes our waterways more than all other industrial sources combined.

- Tremendous amounts of natural resources are consumed and wasted by our modern forms of industrial agriculture: In the United States, 70 percent of all grains, 80 percent of all agricultural land, half of all our water resources, and one-third of all fossil fuels are used to raise animals for food.
- Eating animals destroys the rain forest. Environmentalists now report that the Amazon rain forest has been virtually destroyed to create grazing space for cows. In addition, our rain forests have been devastated to create land where feed is grown for factory-farmed animals, just to supply wealthy nations with meat. A recent report by Greenpeace noted that the chicken-flesh industry, particularly KFC, was primarily responsible for destroying the Amazon.

But the detriment of meat eating is more subtle than all this. Even though the above reasons for vegetarianism are substantial and worthy in their own right, there are horrendous ways in which meat eating affects the consciousness. "Yogis have their own reasons for abstaining from meat," writes Steve Ross, an author and prominent Yoga instructor for more than 20 years. "Yogis don't always look for nourishment first," he continues. "Rather, they look at the vibration of the food." His words are potent:

> When I say *vibration*, I'm referring to the source of the food, and the attitude and the intention of the person preparing it. First Yogis consider the growers of the food. Are the farmers full of gratitude and love, and do they enjoy growing food, or are they angry and filled with hate for their job and all vegetables? These farmers handle the food, and the Yogis believe that their feelings, or vibration, go into the food and thus go into your body if you eat it. Next, Yogis consider the cook. [They, too] affect the vibration, and food can be *poisoned* by a bitter cook.[18]

Ross's most important point, in the present context, is this: "Yogis believe that animals possess consciousness, and therefore to kill them and eat them is to put the energy of fear and violence in the body, because that is the emotional experience of the animal as it dies."[19]

This is a pan-Hindu idea. Writing on behalf of the entire Indic world, including those who practice Yoga, the late *Hinduism Today* guru, Satguru Shivaya Subramuniyaswami, explains the underpinnings of vegetarianism for the spiritually sensitive:

> [Yogis] teach vegetarianism as a way to live with a minimum of hurt to other beings, for to consume meat, fish, fowl or eggs is to participate indirectly in acts of cruelty and violence against the animal kingdom. The abhorrence of injury and killing of any kind leads quite naturally to a

vegetarian diet, sakahara [which is the Sanskrit word for vegetarianism].
The meat-eater's desire for meat drives another to kill and provide that
meat. The act of the butcher begins with the desire of the consumer.
Meat-eating contributes to a mentality of violence, for with the chemically
complex meat ingested, one absorbs the slaughtered creature's fear, pain and
terror. These qualities are nourished within the meat-eater, perpetuating the
cycle of cruelty and confusion. When the individual's consciousness lifts
and expands, he will abhor violence and not be able to even digest the meat,
fish, fowl and eggs he was formerly consuming. India's greatest saints have
confirmed that one cannot eat meat and live a peaceful, harmonious life.
Man's appetite for meat inflicts devastating harm on Earth itself, stripping
its precious forests to make way for pastures. The Tirukural candidly states,
"How can he practice true compassion who eats the flesh of an animal to
fatten his own flesh? Greater than a thousand ghee offerings consumed in
sacrificial fires is not to sacrifice and consume any living creature."[20]

Thus, a true Yogi practices vegetarianism for numerous reasons—not
only because of the importance of *ahimsa* in Patanjai's text or because
the greatest Yoga masters of all time have clearly said that one must be a
vegetarian to advance in Yoga practice. They adopt a vegetarian diet,
too, because their natural sensitivities, which emerge while cultivating
the mode of goodness—something that naturally occurs through the
practice of Yoga—dictate that they do so. It's almost as if they have no
choice: As their consciousness becomes steady—which is one of Yoga's
chief goals: to cease the fluctuations of the mind (*chitta vritti nirodah*)—
they naturally develop compassion for all living beings, and ahimsa manifests as an inescapable way of life.

As an addendum, perhaps, one can even see a respect for creation, specifically for the animal world, in many Yogic *asanas* (postures), so essential
in the practice of Yoga. The interrelation of Yoga and the various creatures
of the world can be traced to ancient Indus Valley seals and shamanic rituals that are all but lost. These led to the adoption of animal *asanas* in
Yoga, with the goal of realigning man's relationship to nature, not least
to the animal world. Both the *Hatha Yoga Pradipika* and the *Gheranda
Samhita*, traditional guidebooks for practice, reveal numerous such *asanas*:
Gomukha-asana ("cow's head pose"), *Kurma-asana* ("turtle's pose"),
Mayur-asana ("peacock's pose"), Simha-asana ("lion's pose")—the crow's
pose, the rooster pose, the cobra pose, the frog pose, the scorpion pose,
and on and on. As Chris Chapple writes:

By imitating an animal, one takes on a new demeanor, influenced by the
qualities of the animal whose shape and form and stance one emulates. In
the performance of the Peacock pose, [for example,] one feels a sense of

balance, pride, an affirmation of one's ability to move competently in the world. ... The strong karmic stance espoused in the tradition of India creates a worldview conducive to animal protection, as seen in the many animal shelters of India and the advocacy of vegetarianism, particularly in the Jain and Vaisnava traditions.[21]

In this way, the numerous animal *asanas* seek to create empathy for animals and the natural world. Such feelings of oneness and camaraderie preclude killing. Thus, even in these *asanas* one finds an implicit statement against harming, torturing or eating animals of any kind.

CONCLUSION

So why would educated Yoga teachers decry vegetarianism, saying that it's okay to eat meat? First of all, I would wager that most are simply uninformed, that is, they really don't know what the tradition has to say about the subject. They are merely people who have become expert in breathing exercises and Yogic postures—"posturing" as people who know Yoga when in fact they do not.

Others may know the texts and the tradition, but they interpret them in erroneous ways. For example, some may say that *ahimsa*, nonviolence, was never meant to include animals. It was only meant as a way to interact with other humans. This is reminiscent of many contemporary reactions to the "thou shalt not kill" commandment in the Judeo-Christian tradition, wherein it is said that the "killing" in this verse only applies to humans. Whatever the case may be in regard to the biblical command— and people do debate its vegetarian implications to the present day—it is quite another matter when it comes to Patanjali's *sutras*. The immediate commentators are clear that it refers to "all violence at all times," and the prominent Yogic authorities, both in days of yore and today, read it like this. The larger tradition was equally clear: vegetarianism is part of the ahimsa sensibility, and aspiring spiritualists were, and are, obliged to give up the eating of meat.

But, in the modern world, the answer is probably a lot more mundane than all this. It is simply about the commodification of spirituality, the degradation of all things profound, the compromise of quality.

Yoga, as is well known, is an increasingly visible and profitable phenomenon in the United States and European health market. No one debates whether its origins or context are found in Vedic India, with its spiritual purpose linked to the tradition commonly known as Hinduism. But few really care. In its popular, widespread incarnation in the modern world, it is not usually learned at the feet of a bona fide guru, but at exercise centers and gyms—or at "Yoga studios." And those who do learn at the feet of a master will likely find themselves involved with a "hodge-podge" master, or one who combines various techniques and who is not herself actually affiliated with a legitimate *sampradaya*, or lineage. This makes for big business.

Yoga, of course, does not have a monopoly on commercialization and commodification. We in the West have witnessed, for example, the recent fate of Christianity. For decades now, we've been subjected to Christian rock groups, bumper stickers, mass-market novels, blockbuster movies, the commercialization of Christmas, and countless other trivializing accoutrements of a compromised tradition. With such mainstream appropriations of an established religious tradition, the practices of its originators fall into oblivion, giving way to more user-friendly versions for people in general. Accordingly, vegetarian Christians are few and far between, though the practice of eschewing a meat-centered diet was common among the religion's founding fathers.[22]

A similar phenomenon now occurs in the Yoga marketplace, making it a commodity, consumable by the masses. Though originally time-honored and deeply profound, these Eastern practices have been repackaged and sold as moderately spiritual alternatives to Western exercise regimens. To make this happen, Yoga was recreated with a de-emphasis on its religious trappings—sometimes consciously but often unconsciously—and gradually became a good way to keep in shape. Period. Special attention, for example, was given to the *asanas*—though this was never Patanjali's emphasis. Rather he gave a special place to *Ishvara-pranidhana*, or devotion to God. But you don't hear much about this in your average Yoga studio. Nor do you hear about the plight of animals or how a Yogi should cultivate compassion for them. Indeed, the Yoga tradition, codified by Patanjali, is now commodified in the West, and few suffer for it as much as the animals.

NOTES

1. The Yoga Site (Yoga Now: Survey Response Data): See http://www.yogasite.com/surveydata.htm.

2. This is slightly down from a 2005 study conducted by the Harris Interactive Service Bureau (HISB), showing that 16.5 million people practice yoga in America.

3. George Feuerstein argues that Vajrayana Buddhism, a form of Tantra Yoga, is one of the few Yogic sects that endorse meat eating, and this, he writes, is largely because of geographical considerations—the mountainous land of Tibet, where this tradition is commonly practiced, does not lend itself to crop cultivation. Otherwise, few Yoga groups would actually encourage meat eating.

See George Feuerstein, *The Deeper Dimension of Yoga* (London: Shambhala, 2003), p. 207.

4. Swami Vivekananda (1863–1902) and Swami Yogananda (1893–1952) are also important contributors to the modern Yoga landscape. Vivekananda is sometimes credited with having brought the practice to Western shores, having authored the book *Raja Yoga*, and Yogananda, with his popular *Autobiography of a Yogi*, made it a public phenomenon. While Yogananda was clearly a supporter of vegetarianism (See *Conversations with Yogananda*, by Swami Kriyananda [Nevada City, California: Crystal Clarity Publishers, 2004, p. 163]), Vivekananda was not. Although the latter spoke about the harmony of all beings and the spiritual oneness of all God's creatures, he was also known to speak out in favor of meat eating. Both he and his teacher, Ramamkrishna, were fish eaters, too—a common practice in his native Bengal—and come from a tradition of Shaktism, which favored animal sacrifice.

With that as background, Vivekananda did write, "All liking for fish and meat disappears when pure Sattva is highly developed, and these are the signs of its manifestation in a soul: sacrifice of everything for others, perfect non-attachment to lust and wealth, want of pride and egotism. The desire for animal food goes when these things are seen in a man" (*Complete works*, 5.403).

5. Brihat Patel, *Krishnamacharya and the Yoga Tradition* (New York: Belis Press, 2007).

6. See http://blog.atmajyoti.org/2009/03/swami-sivananda-on-vegetarian-diet/.

7. See his article "Why be a Vegetarian?" (http://www.liveyourquest.com/E-why_be_a_vegetarian.html).

8. Sharon Gannon, *Yoga and Vegetarianism* (San Rafael, California: Mandala, 2008), p. 26.

9. B. K. S. Iyengar, *Light on Yoga* (New York: Schocken Books, 1966), p. 32.

10. Ibid., p. 37.

11. The general tenor of the earliest texts on vegetarianism and Yoga is perhaps best summed up in the Mahabharata: "Nonviolence is the highest duty" (*ahimsa paro dharmo*). This Sanskrit phrase was popularized by Mahatma Gandhi to demonstrate the universality of nonviolence. It originally comes from the great epic, however, where it is mentioned several times for emphasis. (See especially Anushashana-parvan 116.41.)

12. Accordingly, *ahimsa* is the first precept in the *Hatha Yoga Pradipika* as well: "Nonviolence (*ahimsa*), truth, non-stealing, continence (being absorbed in a pure state of consciousness), forgiveness, endurance, compassion, humility, moderate diet and cleanliness are the ten rules of conduct (*yama*)." See Yogi Swatmarama, *Hatha Yoga Pradipika* (Swami Satyananda Saraswati, Bihar School of Yoga, 1998), p. 56.

13. Gannon, op. cit., pp. 54–69.

14. Ibid., pp. 70–76.

15. See Edwin F. Bryant, *The Yoga Sutras of Patanjali* (New York: North Point Press, 2009), pp. 244–245.

16. For Lord Krishna's explanation of the three modes of nature and their relation to food, see *Bhagavad Gita*, Chapter 17.

17. B. K. S. Iyengar, op. cit., p. 37.

18. Steve Ross, *Happy Yoga* (New York: HarperCollins, 2003), p. 109.

19. Ibid.

20. See Satguru Shivaya Subramuniyaswami, *Dancing With Siva: Hinduism's Contemporary Catechism* (Concord, California: Himalayan Academy, 1993), p. 201.

21. Christopher Key Chapple, *Yoga and the Luminous: Patanjali's Spiritual Path to Freedom* (New York: State University of New York Press, 2008), especially pp. 49 & 56.

22. There are numerous books on vegetarianism and the early Christian tradition. Most thorough, perhaps, are Andrew Linzey, *Animal Theology* (Illinois: University of Illinois Press, 1995); Steven H. Webb, *On Gods and Dogs: A Christian Theology of Compassion for Animals* (New York: Oxford University Press, 1998); and Kerry S. Walters and Lisa Portmess, eds., *Religious Vegetarianism* (New York: State University of New York Press, 2001).

3

Ahimsa in the Patanjali Yoga Tradition[1]

Edwin Bryant

ahimsa paramo dharma—
"Nonviolence is the highest duty"
(*Mahabharata, Vana parva* 207.74; *Drona parva* 192.38)

Like other sacrificial cultures of the ancient world, many of them based on
traditions that continue into the present day, Vedic India's earliest attested
religious practices were centered on highly ritualized oblations that
included the slaughter and offering of animals into the sacred fire. Where
the Indian case is noteworthy and unique in mainstream world religiosity,
is that in the late Vedic period (with stirrings as early as the earlier *Sama
Veda* itself[2]), a strong ethic of *ahimsa*, that is, nonviolence in general, and
vegetarianism in particular, emerged, especially in the ascetic soteriological
traditions (see Bryant, 2006 for discussion[3]).

One of the most important manuals of this genre, which has by now
become a classic in world spirituality, is the *Yoga Sutras of Patanjali*. This
paper examines the role of *ahimsa* in Patanjali's text and its derivative
commentarial tradition.

In 2.30 of the *Yoga Sutras*, after Patanjali first presents the eight limbs of
yoga, we find the following verse:

ahimsa-satyasteya-brahmacaryaparigraha yamah

"The *yamas* are: nonviolence; truthfulness; refraining from stealing; celibacy
and renunciation of [unnecessary] possessions."

In traditional (*Mimamsa*) hermeneutics,[4] introductory (and concluding) statements carry more weight than other statements in scripture.[5]

By this principle, then, say the commentators, *ahimsa*, as the most important of the five *yamas* (the common denominator of which is how one
interacts with other beings), leads the list. Vyasa, the primary commentator on the *Sutras*, accordingly takes *ahimsa* as the root of the other *yamas*.
The *yamas*, by extension, as first on the list of the eight limbs of Yoga, are
in turn the most important ingredient of the entire system, that is, of *Yogic*
practice. Put differently, one's *Yogic* practice remains unsuccessful until
ahimsa is put into practice and perfected.

The goal of the other *yamas* is to achieve *ahimsa* and enhance it, says
Vyasa, and he quotes an unidentified verse stating that one continues to
undertake more and more vows and austerities for the sole purpose of purifying *ahimsa*. Just as the footprints of an elephant cover the footprints of all
other creatures, says Vijnanabhikshu (famous commentator on Patanjali's
Yoga Sutra, flourished in the fifteenth century), so does *ahimsa* cover all
the other *yamas*. As will be touched upon below, the preeminence of
ahimsa is fairly evident in a wide variety of textual traditions.

Vyasa defines *ahimsa* as not injuring any living creature anywhere at any
time. One must strive to avoid harming even an insect as far as possible.[6]
Here he resonates with Manu, the composer of the primary *Dharma Shastra*,
law book, in classical India, who states: "to protect living creatures one
should inspect the ground constantly as one walks, by night or day,
because of the risk of grievous bodily harm" (6.69). Certain ascetic communities, most notably the Jains, still to this day take this at face value
(see Chapple, in this volume). Certainly, one can be very clear about the
fact that eating meat, nourishing one's body at the expense of the suffering
of other living beings, is completely taboo for aspiring *Yogis*. One should
avoid harming even trees, says the commentator Hariharananda.

Ahimsa must be followed in thought, deed and word, says Shankara.
The degree of violence in an act (and hence consequent reaction that
accrues from the action) is determined by intent—acts of violence performed without malice or hatred by a normal person, adds Hariharananda,
such as self-defense, or cutting grass, is not the same as murdering one's
parents in cold blood. But *Yogis* even avoid retaliating in self-defense
against an attacker, he says, and will shoo off a snake rather than kill it,
and thus attempt to inflict as little aggression as possible on their environ-
ments. Nonviolence, Hariharananda continues, also encompasses giving
up the spirit of malice and hatred, since such characteristics result in the
tendency to injure others. This includes avoiding violence in the form of
harsh words, or causing fear in others.

Vyåsa illustrates the primacy of *ahimsa* amongst the *yamas* with a story
indicating that, in the event of conflict between the *yamas*—if observing
one *yama* such as, for example, *satya*, truthfulness, results in the

compromise of another—then *ahimsa* must always be respected as primary. In other words, the other *yamas* are subservient to *ahimsa*, so observing truthfulness, and so on, must never be at the expense of causing harm to others. He relates a narrative from the *Mahabharata* epic of an honest man who is asked by robbers if merchants they are pursuing had passed his way. Since he had seen them do so, and with the second *yama* of *satya* in mind, the man replies truthfully. However, although observing the *yama* of truth, his compliance with the robbers resulted in harm, *himsa*, being caused to the merchants when they were caught as a result of his disclosure. His transgression of the primary ethical injunction thus should have outweighed his observance of the one he chose to follow. Hariharananda applies this principle on a psychological level: if speaking the truth causes distress to another, then *ahimsa* includes not necessarily always bluntly speaking honestly to people about their shortcomings. Here he follows Manu's injunction that "one should not tell the truth unkindly" (4.138).

At the time of writing my *Yoga Sutras* commentary to this verse, there was an ongoing discussion in certain quarters of the Yoga community in the United States about the jurisdiction of the *yamas* in the twenty-first-century West. Relevant to this concern, the next verse of the *Sutras* states:

jati-desha-kala-samayanavacchinnah sarva-bhauma maha-vratam

"[These *yamas*] are considered the great vow. They are not to be abrogated, regardless of one's class, or because of place, time or circumstance. They are universal." (2.31)

In this very important *sutra*, Patanjali states that the *yamas* are absolute and unconditional for aspiring *Yogis*—they cannot be transgressed or exempted under any circumstance such as class (*jati*); place (*desha*); time (*kala*); or circumstance (*samaya*). It is nonnegotiable for *Yogis*. Patanjali is being conspicuously and uncharacteristically emphatic here. There is no sense of dogmaticism in the *Sutras*, much less of any moralizing or proselytizing; this verse is conspicuous in that it is the only verse that has an emphatic or absolutist quality about it.

Clearly, Patanjali is underscoring its significance in the Yogic system: not only are the *yamas* a *vrata*, a vow, but a *mahavrata*, or "great vow." This great vow is further qualified as being *sarva bhauma*, "universal." The term "universal" by definition should make any further qualification redundant—and the very nature of *sutra* writing not only eschews redundancy, but goes to sometimes extreme lengths to condense and compact essential information to the extent of unintelligibility (thereby making most *sutra* study dependent on commentary). Hence, that Patanjali makes a point of additionally naming and eliminating any possible grounds or pleas for exception, despite having already stated that they are absolute, is highly uncharacteristic and therefore significant: these *yamas* are *anavicchinah*, "not to be abrogated," because of one's "class (*jati*); place (*desha*); time (*kala*); or circumstance (*samaya*)," as already mentioned. This is as absolute a statement as can be made.

Therefore, whatever direction the discussions pertaining to the role of the *yamas* in the modern West may take, and whatever hybrid practices evolve in the West under the rubric of *Yoga*, this *sutra* makes it very clear that as far as Patanjali is concerned, for anyone aspiring to be a *Yogi* as defined by his system there are no exceptions to these rules at any time, in any place, for any reason. One might envision that in Patanjali's own circle, there would have been followers or disciples angling for exceptions to one or other of the *yamas*—perhaps arguing that the sacred Vedic law books, the *Dharma Shastras*, themselves allow the *Brahmin* caste, for example, to offer animals in Vedic sacrifices, or the *Kshatriya* caste to eat meat, and so on (we will return to this important dichotomy below). He is therefore being as clear and emphatic here as the straightforward use of human language allows.

One might add that these *yamas* are more-or-less universal amongst all the soteriological (liberation-based) spiritual traditions of ancient India, and even in the more worldly *Dharma Shastra* traditions, the Vedic law books that concern themselves with more worldly socio-civic duties (e.g., Manu 10.63). This is so not only in "orthodox" Vedic traditions (e.g., The *Nyaya Sutras* acknowledge *Yoga* as the means to realize the *atman*, but specify that it entails the following of *yama* and *niyama* ([4.2.45–46]), but "heterodox" traditions too.

The noble eightfold path of Buddhism, for example, requires the observance of four *shilas*, or vows, four of which—*ahimsa*, *satya*, *brahmacharya* and *ashteya*—are identical to the first four *yamas* (one, abstinence from intoxication, replaces *aparigraha*, noncoveting). The Jains, too, have five great vows, for which they use the same term we find here in this *sutra*, *mahavrata*, "great vows," and these are identical to Patanjali's *yamas*.[7] With certain nonmainstream exceptions such as the *Tantric* "left-handed" practices (see Huberman in this volume),[8] these *yamas* are more-or-less standard across Indic sectarian traditions, even if not listed in the specific format chosen by Patanjali. The *Bhagavad Gita*, for example, lists some of the *yamas* in its description of the "divine attributes" (e.g., *ahimsa* and *satya* 16.2); elsewhere in its description of the qualities of *sattva* (e.g., *brahmacharya* and *satya* in 17.14–15); elsewhere in its prescriptions for the *Yogi* (e.g., *aparigraha* in 6.10); and elsewhere again under qualities emanating from Krishna himself (e.g., *brahmacharya* and *satya* X.4–5), and so on.

The commentators elaborate on the conditions listed in this *sutra* through a discussion of nonviolence, since it is the most important *yama* and, as the first member of the list, represents the others (however, the following discussion holds true for all the *yamas*). The *yama* of nonviolence conditioned by caste, says Vyasa, can be seen in the case of, say, a fisherman who, because of his caste occupation inflicts violence only on fish but nowhere else. *Kshatriyas*, the warrior class, too, are allowed to engage in violence in certain contexts—hunting, for example, and, of course, on the battlefield.

While this may hold true in other circumstances, nonviolence has no conditions for Patanjali: *jati* literally means family of birth; therefore, being born into a family or caste that engages in violence or eats meat does not constitute an exception to the practice of nonviolence. In other words, if, say, a *Kshatriya* wishes to become a *Yogi* as understood by Patanjali, he must abandon violence even if such violence is otherwise legitimate for persons of this caste and, indeed, even if it is condoned or even required for that caste by *dharmic* prescriptions in the *Dharma Shastra* texts noted above, which are also considered authoritative as sacred scripture. Manu, for example, who wrote one such law-book, states: "[K]ings who try to kill one another in battle and fight to their utmost ability, never averting their faces, go to heaven" (7.89ff). There would have been spiritual seekers in Patanjali's entourage who would have been coming from *Kshatriya* or other *jatis* who might have pointed to such passages in sacred scripture.

Herein we see a distinction between the requirements of *Yoga* covered in, for example, the *Karma-yoga* section of the *Gita*, where Krishna exhorts Arjuna to do his civic duty as a *Kshatriya* warrior and fight, that is, to specifically engage in violent activity, and the ascetic tradition represented by Patanjali. What may be acceptable or, more, required, in a socio-civic (*dharma*) context must be renounced in an ascetic *Yogic* one. Pursuing this consideration somewhat, one can make a distinction here between *dharma-shastra* and *moksha-shastra* (sacred texts concerning themselves with socio-civic and liberation related prescriptions respectively[9]). What might be appropriate or even prescribed for the former, might be proscribed or forbidden in the latter. Indeed, it is with this ascetic alternative in mind that Arjuna initially wishes to renounce violence and take up the ascetic life of mendicancy so as to pursue the path of nonviolence (2.5). There are numerous instances where we can even find this tension within the pages of the same texts such as the *dharma-shastras* of Manu (see Bryant, previous citation, for discussion).

The *Gita*, of course, while accepting the Patanjalian path of meditation (*Dhyana-yoga*) as an acceptable means to attain liberation (e.g., Chapter Six), has, as part of its agenda, a different objective, one directed to

socio-civic concerns (although everything in the text ultimately culminates in *bhakti*). As both a *dharma-shastra* text and a *moksha-shastra* one,
it is in many ways unique in its construction of a means to attain *moksha*,
liberation from within the parameters and prescriptions of the idealized
social system centered on the upholding of *dharma*, most often referred
to as *Karma-yoga*, "the path of *dharmic* action" (but more commonly
referred to in the text as *Buddhi-yoga* emphasizing its *jnana*, that is, *atma-*
centered, component[10]). While Yoga scholar Whicher (1998, 1999, 2005
and elsewhere) has long argued persuasively that the *Yoga Sutras* too
are not incompatible with social and civic engagement in the world—that
is, once *avidya*, ignorance, is eliminated one can act in the world from a
position of enlightenment[11]—Patanjali's position on the role of the *yamas*
at least, could not be made much clearer. *Tout court*, they are absolute prerequisites for anyone interested in the ultimate goal of life, liberation.

As an example of nonviolence conditioned by place, *desha*, the second
qualifying condition listed in this verse, Vyasa points to a person who
abstains from injury only when in a sacred place, but kills animals elsewhere. Nonviolence must be upheld in all places, he teaches, that is, irrespective of the ritualistic or culinary practices of a particular country or
geographical place. He defines nonviolence conditioned by time, *kala*, as
when one abstains from violence on certain calendar occasions (for example, during religious observations, such as, in a Catholic context, abstaining from meat at Lent), but not at other times. *Yogis* must be nonviolent
at all times.

Finally, nonviolence conditioned by circumstance, *samaya*, the last on
the list, can be exemplified by a person who avoids violence on all occasions except in the context of religious rites. We can recall that the ancient
Vedic *yajna* sacrificial rites, which were still the mainstream religious practices of Patanjali's time, included the ritual offering of animals into the
sacred fire; thus there are prescriptions involving violence in the sacrificial
context outlined in the ancient Vedic texts.[12] Vyasa also gives the example
of soldiers who engage in violence in the context of the battlefield, but
nowhere else, as we have illustrated with Arjuna above. Under *samavaya*,
one might also mention allowances made in *Ayurveda*, the traditional
Hindu system of medicinal knowledge, for temporarily imbibing certain
meat substances to cure certain very specific medical conditions.

In short, even if one's very *dharma*, righteous duty, allows for or even
prescribes exceptions to *ahimsa* based on *jati*, *kala*, *desha*, or *samavaya*, if
one wishes to be a *Yogi*, such conditions or exceptions no longer apply.
All these exceptions may be legitimate or valid elsewhere in other contexts
but, for the *Yogi* wishing to attain the goals of *Yoga* outlined in this text, say
the commentators, this *sutra* very emphatically specifies that any such

mitigating factors or conditions no longer apply; nonviolence and the other *yamas* must be practiced at all times, in all conditions, everywhere, irrespective of any considerations whatsoever. One can take this or leave it, but Patanjali's intent cannot be expressed much more clearly. Again, the *yamas* are universal prescriptions—there are no exceptions, says Vyasa. Aspiring *Yogis* in the modern context are thus informed in this *sutra* that renegotiations of the *yamas* due to the exigencies of modern times and the western landscape are emphatically not recognized by the classical Yoga tradition. Hence Patanjali states that the *yamas* are the "universal great vow."

What, then, is an aspiring *Yogi* to do if, by the force of past habits, cultural upbringing or even religious commandment, the craving or impulse to eat meat arises in the mind (*chitta*)? Here we must introduce the notion of *samskara*. *Samskaras* are a very important feature of *Yoga* psychology: every sensual experience or mental thought that has ever been experienced forms a *samskara*, an imprint, in the *chitta* mind, before fading away, like a sound is imprinted on a CD, or an image in a camera. The mind is thus a storehouse of these recorded *samskaras*, deposited and accumulated in the *chitta* over countless lifetimes. Memories, in Hindu psychology, are considered to be vivid *samskaras* from this lifetime, which are retrievable, while the notion of the subconscious in Western psychology corresponds to other less retrievable *samskaras*, perhaps from previous lives, which remain latent as subliminal impressions. *Samskaras* also account for such things as personality traits, habits, cravings, impulses, compulsive and addictive behaviors, and so on. For example, a particular type of experience, say eating meat, is imprinted in the *chitta* as a *samskara*, which then activates as a desirable memory or impulse provocation, triggering a repetition of this activity, which is likewise recorded, and so on until a cluster or groove of *samskaras* of an identical or similar sort is produced in the *chitta*, gaining strength with each repetition. The stronger or more dominant such a cluster of *samskaras* becomes, the more it activates regularly and imposes itself upon the consciousness of the individual, demanding indulgence and perpetuating a vicious cycle that can be very hard to break. So what does *Yoga* prescribe for an aspiring *Yogi*, who, despite being committed to a more enlightened and compassionate relationship with other beings, is still afflicted with a craving for flesh due to such *samskaras* of previous indulgence? With this in mind, in the next two verses, Patanjali states:

vitarka-bandhane pratipaksha-bhavanam//vitarka himsadayah krita-karitanumodita-lobha-krodha-moha-purvaka mridu-madhyadhimatra duhk-hajnanananta-phala iti pratipaksha-bhavanam

"Upon being harassed by negative thoughts, one should cultivate counteracting thoughts. Negative thoughts are violence, etc. They may be [personally] performed, performed on one's behalf by another, or authorized by oneself; they may be triggered by greed, anger, or delusion; and they may be slight, moderate or extreme in intensity. One should cultivate counteracting thoughts, because the end results [of negative thoughts] are ongoing suffering and ignorance." (2.33–34)

"Negative thoughts," *vitarkas*, are defined here by Patanjali as being thoughts countering the *yamas* such as *ahimsa*, that is, thoughts directed towards violence, untruthfulness, and so on. The craving to eat meat is thus a *vitarka*. It is important to note here, and aspiring *Yogis* might be reassured to do so, that Patanjali has specified here "when" one is afflicted by *vitarkas*, not "if." How can such thoughts not arise? They are simply the cropping up of *samskaras*, present in great abundance in the *chittas* of all entities, past indulgences or cruel behaviors that all embodied beings have performed at some point just by dint of being subject to the ever-changing *gunas*. They *will* tend to surface until the *Yogi* is very advanced and has burnt up the productive power of all latent *samskaras* by the force of Yogic practice. The task, then, is not to become despondent upon their periodic and inevitable emergence, nor berate oneself when they arise, but to counter them in the manner outlined here.

A deeper understanding of the process underpinning the workings of the mind (*chitta*), which, one must always keep in mind, is considered a material (*prakritic*) entity in Yoga and not an aspect of the soul (*atman/purusha*), requires the introduction of a further set of categories: the three *gunas*, "strands" or "qualities." Metaphysically, the mind is essentially composed of three *gunas*: *sattva*, "lucidity"; *rajas*, "action"; and *tamas*, "inertia."[13] *Sattva*, the purest of the *gunas* when manifested in the *chitta*, is typically characterized, amongst a number of things, by lucidity, compassion, tranquility, wisdom, discrimination, detachment, happiness, and peacefulness; *rajas*, by hankering, energetic endeavor, power, and restlessness and all forms of movement and creative activity; and *tamas*, the *guna* least favorable for *Yoga*, by ignorance, delusion, disinterest, lethargy, sleep, and disinclination toward constructive activity. The *Bhagavad Gita* (Chapters 14, 17, and 18) presents a wide range of symptoms connected with each of these three *gunas*.[14] Krishna makes the useful observation that the *gunas* are in continual tension with each other, one *guna* becoming prominent in an individual for a while and suppressing the others, only to be dominated in turn by the emergence of one of the other *gunas* (*Bhagavad Gita* 14.10).

One of the goals of *Yoga* meditation, as discussed repeatedly in the traditional literature, is to maximize the presence of *sattva guna* in one's mind and minimize that of *rajas* and *tamas*. According to Samkhya metaphysics, all three *gunas* are inherently present in all the material byproducts of *prakriti*, including the *chitta*, so *rajas* and *tamas* can never be eliminated, merely minimized or, at best, reduced to a latent and unmanifest potential. Clearly, *sattva* is the *guna* most conducive, indeed, indispensable, to the *Yogic* enterprise. But while *rajas* and *tamas* are universally depicted as obstacles to *Yoga*, a certain amount of each *guna* is indispensable to embodied existence. (Without *tamas* for example, there would be no sleep, and without *rajas* no digestion or even the energy to blink an eyelid.) Even so, *Yoga* is overwhelmingly about cultivating or maximizing *sattva*. Another way of putting this, is that *sattva* should control whatever degree of *rajas* and *tamas* are indispensable to healthy survival—sleeping for 6 or 7 hours, for example, rather than 10, eating a modest amount of food, rather than gorging, and so on. *Samskaras*, then—desires, thoughts, memories, habits, patterns of behavior—as products of the mind, can be either *sattvic*, *rajasic*, or *tamasic*.

Like weeds in even the best-tended of gardens, the *vitarkas*, or unwanted thoughts of this verse—which we can now categorize as *rajasic* or *tamasic samskaras*—inevitably emerge from time to time. As indicated in the *Gita*: "One in whom all desires flow by [but who remains undisturbed by them] like the ocean into which the rivers flow but which remains undisturbed, attains peace" (2.70); and, again, "one who neither begrudges or hankers for the presence or absence of lucidity, activity or delusion [*sattva*, *rajas* and *tamas*], but who remains as if indifferent, and is not disturbed by the *gunas* thinking 'the *gunas* alone are operating' ... is said to have transcended the *gunas*" (14.22–25). Desires will crop up; *rajas* and *tamas* will manifest in the *chitta*; *vitarkas* such as thoughts of *himsa* will emerge from our subconscious or conscious minds. Hence, Patanjali implies in this *sutra* that the task is not to berate oneself upon contemplating a "negative thought," such as *himsa*, but to deal with such occurrences insightfully. This, according to Patanjali, means "considering their consequences" (*pratipakshbhavana*).

The *vitarkas*, that is, thoughts of violence and so on, contrary to the *yamas* are divided into three categories by Patanjali: those one actually performs oneself, *krita*; those that one has others perform on one's behalf, *karita*; and those that one approves of or authorizes in some way, *anumodita*. So, killing an animal oneself would come under the first category; purchasing meat which has been killed by someone else, in the second category; and allowing meat consumption to occur in one's sphere of influence, even if one does not consume the meat oneself, would come under the third category. This resonates with Manu: "The one who gives permission [to eat meat], the one who butchers, the one who slaughters, the one who buys and sells, the one who prepares, the one who serves, and the

eater—they are all killers" (5.51).[15] The Buddha, too, made a similar
statement: "Monks, one possessed of three qualities is put into Hell
according to his deserts. What three? One who is himself a taker of life,
encourages another to do the same, and approves thereof."[16]

Patanjali is being fairly specific here, says Bhoja Raja, otherwise some
"dull-wit" (as he puts it) may think that since the violence involved in killing the animal was performed by someone else, the actual eater of the
meat avoids *karmic* responsibilities. Vijnanabhikshu includes here even
violence condoned in the scriptures, viz., that animals can be killed and
eaten under certain conditions or according to religious regulatory prescriptions (such as in the context of Vedic sacrifice or other religiously
specified acts of slaughter). Hariharananda goes further and rejects the
idea that God has allowed certain types of animal consumption. The emergence of a vegetarian ethic such as that expressed here and in most post-
Vedic Hinduism from the matriarchal culture of ritual slaughter inherent
in the ancient Vedic sacrificial texts is an interesting phenomenon which
I have examined elsewhere.[17]

Each of these categories, continues Vyasa, have been further subdivided
into three degrees of intensity by Patanjali—*mridumadhya-adhimatra*,
slight, moderate, or extreme. Additionally, they may be provoked in three
ways: by greed, *lobha*, such as in the case of a person who inflicts violence
on animals out of lust for their meat or with an eye to profit from their
skins; anger, *krodha*, such as in the case of the person who lashes out vio-
lently upon being insulted by someone else; or illusion, *moha*, such as when
one engages in violence under the impression that it is one's duty, or that
it is religiously condoned (as in killing animals in a religious context, says
Vijnanabhikshu).

Since greed, anger, and delusion can underpin acts done oneself, on
one's behalf, or authorized by oneself, *krita-karitanumodita*, and can be
experienced in three degrees of intensity, there are 27 divisions of violence, and so forth, noted by Patanjali in this *sutra*. Characteristic of the
penchant for categorization often found in traditional Indic commentaries[18]
Vyasa trebles this number, bringing the possibilities up to 81.[19] Actually,
continues Vyasa, the possibilities are innumerable since there are other
factors qualifying violence, such as customary rules and other types of
options (Vijnanabhikshu exemplifies "customary rules" as the view that
violence can only be inflicted on fish, not animals, and Vyasa's "other types
of options" as that particular animals can be killed and eaten only on
certain days).

To counter thoughts of this kind, one should cultivate countering
thoughts—thoughts on the consequences of such activities, such as Patanjali's suggestion that violence leads to unlimited suffering and ignorance to

the agent. As a result of the perpetrator of violence first overpowering the helpless animal victim, then inflicting violence on it by weapons, and then taking its life, the perpetrator's own life forces are weakened in this life, says Vyasa. And in the next life, he or she takes birth in hell,[20] or in a lower species of life, where, says Vijnanabhikshu, the very same violence previously inflicted on other creatures is experienced by the perpetrator. By the laws of *karma* (that every action provokes an equal and commensurate reaction) every act of violence inflicted on another entity by a given agent creates a seed of corresponding violence that must be experienced by that same agent as a reaction. This reaction accrues even if, as Patanjali has stressed in these verses, the act of violence was not performed by the agent but on his or her behalf, or even if facilitated by the agent in any way. Hence, Patanjali's statement that inflicting violence eventually brings suffering to the agent.

Violent people live every moment as though dead, Vyasa continues. Indeed, they may even crave death, he writes, but are forced to live on because, by the law of *karma*, some of the mandated fruits of their activities have to be experienced in this life. For example, says Vijnanabhikshu, a person may be tormented by a horrible prolonged disease as a *karmic* consequence of past acts performed by that very person. Even one who is violent appears to experience happiness in this life, notes Vyasa; this is due to good *karmic* reaction accrued from performing pious activities in a past life that are bearing fruits in this one. These good reactions can balance out some of the bad *karmic* reaction from the violence being committed in the present (just as seeds of grain are sown along with seeds of grass, says Vijnanabhikshu), but the negative *karma* will manifest in some other fashion—a short lifespan, for example—or, of course, the seeds of violence being sown in this life may lay dormant until the next life.

By the law of action and reaction, violence always eventually breeds suffering for the perpetrator, who has to personally experience the same sort of violence he or she inflicted on other beings. Violence also breeds ignorance, *ajnana*, the second consequence of perverse thoughts mentioned in these verses by Patanjali. Vachaspati Mishra states that violence is the result of *tamas*, contributing to further *tamas* and perpetuating violence that increases the *tamas*, ignorance, of the *chitta*. Real knowledge of the *atman*, the ultimate true self beyond the *chitta*, is thus further covered over. Due to *tamas*, then, one becomes less likely to ponder the reactions of one's violence or other harmful activities and thus less aware of the *karmic* consequences one is creating for oneself.

Ultimately, all creatures are parts of *Ishvara*, God, adds Vijnanabhikshu, like sons to the father and sparks to the fire. Therefore, violence against others is violence against God. He quotes the *Gita:* "Envious people act hatefully towards me [Krishna] in their own and in others' bodies. I continually hurl such cruel, hateful people, the lowest of mankind, into *samsaric* existences, into only the impure wombs of demons" (16.19).

Thus, reflecting on the undesirable consequences of *vitarkas*, "negative thoughts," in some of these ways, one should not allow the mind to indulge them. When one is tormented by *vitarkas*, says Vyasa, such as: "I will inflict violence," one should cultivate counter thoughts. One should rather think: "Burning in the fire of this world, I have taken shelter of *Yoga* by committing myself to the welfare of all creatures; after having renounced such perverse thoughts, by again resorting to them, I am behaving like a dog who licks its own vomit."

Actually, this *sutra* is profound in its implications, and provides a means of performing a type of mindfulness, whereby one consciously adjusts the types of *samskaras* one allows in one's *chitta*. If we consider the *chitta* to be essentially a warehouse of *samskaras*, the *vitarkas*, negative thoughts, are merely the activation of some of these previous *samskaras* lying in storage; *samskaras* are never destroyed (although they can be "burnt" by *Yogic* practice). In other words, thoughts of violence, arise because of the past practices of such things that are then imprinted on one's *chitta*. If, when the *Yogi* becomes aware of a *himsa*-related thought arising in the *chitta*, he or she makes a conscious effort to counter it by invoking a benevolent thought, then, by doing so, a new, more *sattvic* type of *samskara* is planted in the *chitta* warehouse.

For example, if an aspiring *Yogi* feels a craving for meat, then he or she might contemplate, and even visualize, the suffering inflicted on innocent animals in the process of their slaughter—perhaps by observing the feelings, emotions, and affection exhibited by one's adored and cuddly pets (as the Jains urge us to do) and then projecting these observations onto all other (perhaps not so cuddly) animals. Or, perhaps better for struggling *Yogis* possessed with a relentless sense of moral integrity and brutal truthfulness, force themselves to visit the realities of a slaughterhouse. These experiences will form new *samskaras* that can counteract—do battle with, if you like—the meat-craving *samskaras*.

While the Indic admonitions against violence to animals stem from moral and compassion-derived sensitivities, one might just as well ponder the additional observations promoted by modern Western concerns against meat eating. There are plenty of resources outlining the devastating environmental, economic, or health repercussions of a meat-centered diet. These newly cultivated *sattvic* thoughts, along with reflecting on the negative consequences of perverse thinking, such as the bad *karma* from meat eating accruing to oneself discussed above, are then recorded in the *chitta* as beneficial *samskaras*.

The more one practices this type of benevolent and insightful *sattvic* thinking in opposition to the *rajasic* and *tamasic* thoughts that underpin inclinations towards violence, the more the texture of the *chitta* is transformed from *rajasic* and *tamasic* to *sattvic*. The more the *chitta* becomes "*sattvicized*" in this way, the less frequently *rajasic* and *tamasic* thoughts will surface, and the less effort one will have to make to actually cultivate *sattva* (artificially, so to speak)—*sattvic* thoughts will start to arise more naturally and spontaneously.

As in a garden flowerbed, the more one makes an effort to uproot weeds, the more the bed will eventually become a receptacle for fragrant flowers, which will then grow and reroot or reseed of their own accord until there is hardly any room for weeds to surface. In other words, as *sattva* is cultivated in this way, the personality of the *Yogi* becomes altered. Weeding, of course, can never be abandoned completely, and even the most saintly and accomplished *Yogi* must be ever-vigilant for old *rajasic* and *tamasic samskaras* lying dormant in the subconscious depths of the *chitta*, like the latent seeds of dormant weeds. Hence Patanjali states in 2.31 that *Yogic* practice can never be given up as long as one is embodied. (*Yogis* who accept Patanali as an authority thus steer clear of anyone claiming to have "transcended" the need for following the *yamas*, or renegotiating them in the name of some higher esoteric spiritual principle.)

Cultivating the opposite types of thoughts is the means to remove perverse ideas from the mind. When negative thoughts are eliminated, powers accrue to the *Yogi*. These are indicative of the *Yogi's* success in this regard and are the subject of the next *sutras*, 2.35–45, which conclude Patanjali's comments on *ahimsa*. In this section, Patanjali selects some of the boons that accrue to the *Yogi* by following, *pratishtha*, each of the 10 *yamas* and *niyamas* respectively, beginning, as always, with *ahimsa*.

ahimsa-pratishthayam tat-sannidhau vaira-tyagah

In the presence of one who is established in nonviolence, enmity is abandoned. (2.35)

Vyasa comments on Patanjali's verse here that all living beings give up their enmity in the presence of one who is established in nonviolence. Put differently, a saint exudes qualities that rub off on his or her associates. That is to say, like the halos in Christian art forms, the *Yogi's sattvic* mind can pervade out, and consequently "*sattvicize*" the minds of other beings in the vicinity, countering the *rajas* and *tamas* of others, stimulating their *sattvic* potential. The commentators state that even natural enemies such as the cat and mouse, or mongoose and snake, give up their enmity in the presence of the *Yogi* who has fully given up all thoughts of violence, due to being influenced by the *Yogi's* state of mind. One is reminded here of an episode in the hagiography of the sixteenth-century mystic Chaitanya Mahaprabhu, who caused the deer and tigers in the forest to dance and embrace each other upon hearing him recite the holy names of Krishna.[21] Such accounts surface in numerous traditions: one might mention Saint Francis of Assisi and his taming of the wild wolf, and the Moroccan Sufi women saints, Rabi'a, who lived on a hill surrounded by wild animals,[22] and the furious elephant Nalagiri, who became quiet in the presence of the Buddha.[23]

In conclusion, then, *ahimsa*, as the very first item on the list of the *Yogangas*, "limbs of *Yoga*," is not only an indispensable but also a nonnegotiable preliminary ingredient of spiritual life as prescribed by Patanjali. It is as applicable today as it was two millennia ago in ancient India for those identifying with or even aspiring to be *Yogis* as the term is understood in, not just the *Yoga Sutras*, but almost the entirety of mainstream classical Sanskrit literature in its many genres. Without following *ahimsa*, one cannot claim to be following the *Yoga* of Patanjali or of any other of ancient India's soteriological spiritual traditions.

NOTES

1. Much of the material for this paper has its roots in my recent translation and commentary of Bryant, Edwin F., *The Yoga Sutras of Patanjali* (New York: North Point Press, 2009), pp. 244–245.

2. The oldest Vedic texts are the four Vedas, one of which is the *Sama*, wherein it is stated: "we use no sacrificial stake, we slay no victims, we worship entirely by the repetition of sacred verses" (I.176).

3. "Strategies of Subversion." In *A Communion of Subjects*. Eds., Waldau, P. and Patton, K. (New York: Columbia University Press, 2006), pp. 194–202.

4. Hermeneutics were the specialization of Mimamsa, one of the classical six schools of philosophy.

5. See, for example, Shankara's commentary to the *Vedanta Sutras* 1.1.4.

6. Although *ahimsa* has been defined by Vyasa as not harming any creature anywhere at any time, one must continue to perform one's *dharma*, duty, cautions Vijnanabhikshu, even though it is impossible to avoid harming tiny living entities such as bacteria or insects when one engages in activities such as bathing or cleaning, etc.

7. *Vide Uttaradhyayana* XXIII.12.

8. Certain "left-handed" *Tantric* rites prescribe (highly) ritually circumscribed imbibing of meat or other prohibited substances, including intoxicating substances, along with indulgence in sexual practices with a view to transcending dualistic notions of "purity" and "pollution," and facilitating an experience of the divine interplay underpinning material reality as conceived of in the *Shakta* traditions. But even here, these practices are not performed in a licentious manner,

but with complex ritual and meditational conditions. Right handed *Tantra*, however, tends to observe and promote *yama*-type principles (e.g., *Devi Gita* 5.6).

9. In late Vedic discourse, the goals of life (*purusha-arthas*) are sometimes construed as fourfold: *dharma* (socio-civic duties), *artha* (material prosperity and well-being); *kama* (pursuit of sensual pleasure); and *moksha* (liberation). Each of these has a body of scriptural texts (*shastra*) associated with it.

10. This refers to the *Upanishadic* teaching that the real self is not the body or the mind.

11. More technically, one can act through the *aklishta vrittis*, the states of mind that does not impede the goal of *Yoga* of 1.5, viz., *vrittis* not produced from *kleshas*, impediments, such as *avidya*, ignorance.

12. *Vide* Bryant, "Strategies of Subversion." In *A Communion of Subjects* (2006), referred to previously, for discussion.

13. Although everything in reality, including the physical and cosmological aspect of the universe is also a product of the three *gunas*, the Yoga tradition in interested in their psychic aspect.

14. These cover such things as: prescribed duty and its mode of performance, worship, diet, charity, sacrifice, austerity, knowledge, activity, understanding, determination, attainment of happiness, and future birth. See, also, Manu, 12.24–52.

15. Doniger, Wendy and Smith, Bryan K., trans., *The Laws of Manu* (London: Penguin, 1991), p. 104.

16. *Anguttara Nikaya* 3.17.1.

17. *Vide* Bryant, "Strategies of Subversion." In *A Communion of Subjects*, previous reference.

18. Even in the sparse *Sutras* themselves *mridumadhyadhimatra* occurs again in 1.22.

19. In other words, Vyasa proposes that the intensity of greed, anger, and delusion can be mildly mild, moderately mild, or extremely mild; mildly moderate, moderately moderate, and extremely moderate; and mildly extreme, moderately extreme, and extremely extreme (probably with the set of subdivisions from 1.21–22 in mind)!

20. Hell, in Indic thought, is not a situation of eternal damnation, but a location to which one goes to suffer the fruits of particularly negative *karma*, until such *karma* has been accounted for. One must remain in such locations until one has oneself finished experiencing all the suffering one inflicted upon others when in the human form, after which one may be reborn as a human again. (There have been one or two commentators on the Vedanta, such as Madhva and Vallabha, who interpret the verse from *Gita* quoted by Vijnanabhiksu below, as pointing to a class of entity that is eternally condemned; this, however, is an exceptional view in Hinduism and rarely endorsed.)

21. *Caitanya Caritamrita*, Madhya Lila, 17 37.

22. Rosen, Steven, *Diet for Transcendence: Vegetarianism and the World Religions* (Badger, California: Torchlight Books, 1998), p. 63.

23. *Vinaya Pitaka Cullavagga* 7.8.13.

4

Ashtanga Yoga Body: Feel Your Way to Enlightened Eating

Kino MacGregor

Yoga is a conscious effort to train the mind to be fully present by control-ling the body, breath, and mind in one harmonious moment. The physical postures of Yoga are knit together with careful attention to the breath and the practitioner's point of focus. The physical postures produce the added side effects of cleansing the body, ridding practitioners of unwanted fat, and healing old injuries. By bringing the body and mind deeper into unity, Yoga practitioners naturally develop a peaceful relationship with their environment. One almost-universal way that most Yogis create peace in their lives is by adhering to a diet that does not harm other beings for personal sustenance.

Yoga is not just another form of exercise. Instead, it is a body-awareness technique aimed at liberating one's consciousness from old, habitual ways of thinking, being, and acting. The lithe, flexible Yoga body is merely a seductive by-product of the work of awakening one's consciousness. Although many Yoga practitioners learn that eating a light vegetarian diet is conducive to a daily *asana* practice, the real motivation of Yogis to change their dietary habits is a moral one. The commitment not to do harm, known in Sanskrit as *ahimsa*, forms the basis of the Yoga student's relationship with food. Rather than merely explaining any new lifestyle in terms of physical benefits, the tradition of Yoga always explains new devel-opments in terms of their spiritual goal. The Yoga diet helps students reaffirm their commitment to live a spiritual life with every bite they take.

Nearly 20 million Americans are using their dollars to buy into a new currency of soul by practicing Yoga. While there is at least a popular notion of what Yoga is, the real practice of this ancient modality represents a unique chance to reclaim the true pioneering spirit of the human soul. Whereas the moral dilemma regarding food sources is more common in the spiritual traditions of the East, the choice to move towards a vegetarian diet stakes out new territory in the Western world. In some sense, it is a bold move that must be predicated on years of spiritual practice in order for the decision to take root.

SRI K. PATTABHI JOIS

My teacher, the late Sri K. Pattabhi Jois, taught me the Ashtanga Yoga method in great detail and guided many students, like me, toward a simple vegetarian diet. The perspective presented here comes from a dedicated student of Jois and the Ashtanga Yoga method and is necessarily biased by the daily practice of such an arduous discipline. In order to understand the relationship between the Ashtanga Yoga tradition and any lifestyle changes it asks of practitioners, it is crucial to understand more about the tradition itself. There is much more to Yoga than bending, folding, and twisting your body. Indeed, Yoga also stretches your mind by asking you to challenge your beliefs about yourself, your body, your consciousness, your identity, and your community. In doing so, Yoga creates real and lasting change in the lives of its many practitioners.

The miracle of Jois's life and legacy far exceeds his physical presence and is perhaps the very definition of the word Guru. Born as a Brahmin in a small village called Kowshika in Southern India on Guru Purnima day, the first full moon of July designated in 1915 as a national holiday in India to honor all Gurus, Jois's life embodied the tradition of the sacred teacher-student relationship. Jois was initially a devoted student after discovering Yoga at the age of 12 when he saw the man who would become his teacher, T. Krishnamacharya. He then continued his education in Yoga and Sanskrit at Mysore University until after 37 years of professorship he earned the title of Vidwan (marking him professor emeritus of Sanskrit Studies).

The choice to live a spiritual life was central to his Jois's studies and was necessarily reflected in the traditional dietary choices of a Brahmin in India, that is, a simple vegetarian diet. Jois died when he was 93 years old after dedicating his life to the teaching of Ashtanga yoga, a dynamic flowing series of postures that he introduced to the West nearly 35 years before his passing. With more than 65 years of experience teaching in the small south India city of Mysore, Jois's unwavering diligence in maintaining the Ashtanga Yoga method as he learned it from his teacher, T. Krishnamacharya, allowed thousands if not millions of people to benefit

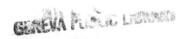

from regular Ashtanga Yoga practice. Without his steady perseverance throughout more than half of the twentieth century, Yoga as we know it today simply would not be.

Ashtanga Yoga traces its lineage to an ancient sage named Vamana Rishi, whose direct line of teachers reached all the way to Jois. Jois' teacher, Krishnamacharya, is known as the source of most of the Yoga that is now popularly taught in the West. His students have developed and taught Iyengar Yoga, Viniyoga, and Ashtanga Yoga.

Krishnamacharya was also famous for teaching Indra Devi, the first female student of Yoga in the larger tradition, only after he demanded that she eat only root vegetables for a long period of time. Krishnamacharya's teacher was Rama Mohan Brahmachari, who lived in a cave in the Himalayas. Lineage in Yoga is much like tracing a family tree. You learn from a teacher who is a student of one master. The master who is your teacher's teacher was once a student of a master as well. So it goes in an unbroken line from teacher to student back through a nearly 5,000-year journey of Indian history. Preserved without the ease of computers, typeface-printing machines, and back-up space on external hard disks, most Yoga knowledge comes from teachers enforcing direct memorization on their students. Deeply ingrained into this sacred tradition is a way of relating to the body, the mind, and the Earth that makes the choice to eat a peaceful diet self-evident.

ASHTANGA YOGA

Ashtanga yoga is broken up into six segments of postures. The first group of postures is called the Primary Series and is a pretty strenuous exercise routine. Most people will spend their entire lives working on elements of this set of 72 postures. It is called Yoga *Chikitsa* and cleanses your physical body, organs, tissues, glands, and fat. Most students of Ashtanga Yoga begin to feel their inner body in a more pronounced way after some time of practicing, so much so that they can actually feel the effects of various food choices directly within themselves. Only then are students really ready to investigate the deeper meaning of evolving their relationship with food.

Ashtanga Yoga asks you to work on the spiritual through the physical. You begin by sweating your way through some Yoga postures while concentrating your mind on your body, breath, and gaze. The Primary Series of Ashtanga Yoga contains all the necessary elements for establishing health and purifying your body. It includes forward bending, twisting, backward bending, lifting, head-standing and the Sun Salutation, or *Surya Namaskara.*

The specific nature of Ashtanga Yoga is that you repeat the same order of postures until you have mastered them. You do not get to move on until you have made some sort of progress where you are. When you repeat a series of postures over and over, you move out of the intellectual understanding and into a kinesthetic intelligence that connects movement to soul. In a sense, the deepening relationship that Ashtanga practitioners make with their bodies demands that they get more attuned to subtle sense perception. It is this refined awareness that allows the transition to a vegetarian diet to take place.

Ashtanga Yoga asks tightness to bend and softness to be strong. It challenges the limits of the mind and the body beyond popular medical notions of safety, possibility, and comfort. In doing so, practitioners literally expand their consciousness. Although Ashtanga Yoga contains six series of postures, most practitioners spend their entire lives working on the first, or Primary Series, because its level of strength and flexibility demands is already quite challenging. Yet the Primary Series is a complete practice that burns through accumulated toxins within the body and heightens the level of health.

Without regular cleansing the body collects toxins from the environment, food, and even emotional states that if left unattended can sometimes lead to disease and discomfort later in life. Once students experience how difficult it can be to remove toxins from the body, they often want to eat and live in such a way that minimizes the addition of toxicity to their bodies. The physical practice of Yoga can be likened to brushing your teeth. Without a daily routine, plaque and tartar accumulate and cause a pricey visit to the dentist. Yet with Yoga, youth, health, and comfort can easily return to the body through proven methods of practice. It is no magic pill, however, for it is through your own effort that you purify your body. Yoga is as strong as you make it and takes you as deep as you are willing to go.

The connection between the physical practice and the spiritual transformation is one of the most mystical experiences in the path of Yoga. No one can quite define exactly how the body, mind, and soul unite in each breath to produce momentous life change. Yet practitioners all around the world experience just that. The high level of difficulty in Ashtanga Yoga combined with the fast-paced order of the postures quiets the mind so dramatically that new thoughts have the space to enter later in the day after practice. The silent space of the Ashtanga Yoga Mysore room does not require philosophy or lifestyle changes by the students but instead allows the Yoga to work in mysterious and sometimes magical ways. Jois never told his students that in order to do Yoga they needed to change their diet or their relationship with food. Instead, he let the Yoga work itself individually through each student. Almost every student of Ashtanga Yoga feels a desire to change their relationship with food because of the inner changes that Yoga stimulates on a deep level.

ASHTANGA YOGA AND DIET

Since Yoga is a body-awareness technique and Ashtanga Yoga asks students to feel their bodies in their entirety, it is the Yoga itself that brings about the request to delve deeper into the students' relationship with that which is good. Although most Yoga students are interested in changing their diets almost from the beginning, Ashtanga Yoga relies on direct experience rather than theory. It is only when the student actually feels the deleterious effects of harmful or unhealthy foods in their own body through the laboratory of their daily Yoga practice that Ashtanga Yoga really considers they are ready to change. Ashtanga Yoga teachers wait for the moment when new Yoga practitioners genuinely want to start deconstructing their kitchens to redirect the students' diets according to the Yogic diet guidelines.

Rather than merely handing new students a list of dietary dos and don'ts, Ashtanga Yoga asks practitioners to go deeper along the path of self-inquiry and develop consciousness around the whole process of food. When new Yoga practitioners simply transplant dietary guidelines onto their lives as though dictated from above, they merely use Yoga to reenact an all-or-nothing mentality that characterizes fad dieting.

Instead, the real path of Yoga asks practitioners to question everything until they know truth firsthand. Food is part of the process of detailed self-inquiry. As such, the journey begins with understanding that food is not who you are. It is a way you communicate with the world. You express things through eating, like you do through any art form, but it nevertheless is not who you are in your deepest essence. Your eating habits are merely habits, not your life or your vitality, though they may seriously affect your life, your energy levels, and your overall health.

If you actually begin to think about this on a material level, food creates your body anew, giving the substance of the meat on your bones. What nutrients you take in, literally become your body. It is a blending and an intimacy perhaps only paralleled by the sexual act. If you begin to think about your eating habits and your food consumption as a sacred act of intimacy between you and the world around you, eating takes on a whole new perspective. You might begin to ask what you actually want inside of you. Your choices about food actually reflect your level of self-esteem. In every morsel that enters your mouth there is a de facto statement about what you think you're worth, that is, what you think is good enough to enter the private or sacred sphere of your body.

Sometimes self-worth is the missing element in one's dietary plan or regime. Often, harsh diets give people with low self-esteem a place to hide their insecurities rather than move through them. Under the severity of dietary regimes, a person with low self-esteem may turn to a diet and mistakenly think that they will become worthy, good, and healthy only by following the strict rules presented before them. In some ways, strict dietary rules are a kind of dependency of the mind. On a deeper level, strictness, tightness, and rigidity around food is a silent and often subliminal statement of the fear of feeling out of control, a cry for help mistakenly placed on something external. This power is inappropriately placed in the food rather than in the being who chooses, consumes, enjoys, and embodies the food.

There is power hidden in our relationship to food. There is a latent potential that rests between each tasty morsel that passes through the space between your lips. The choices you make about food on any given day are a snapshot of your sense of self-worth. Each time you eat, you say yes to a whole way of being, living, and feeling. And each time you eat you also say no to an even wider scope of the world. Eating is an intimacy that when properly honored becomes and evolves into a celebration of your highest potential for health and wellbeing.

Yet you do not always eat for sustenance and optimum health. Sometimes you eat out of pleasure, boredom, habit, guilt, escape, and addiction, to name a few. These emotions and their intricate ties to food can lead to a cycle of negativity and guilt. Sometimes we find ourselves eating without any real consciousness, in a kind of blind and deaf numbness. It is in these moments of oblivion that our choices are often hard to face—because they're often invisible to us. Sometimes the relationship to food can be colored by the cycle of craving, addiction, and disorder. And yet it is in these very destructive patterns that ultimately give you access to your greatest source of transformation.

Although it may not always seem like it, that which you say yes to is entirely up to you. You are the one responsible for all your choices in life and especially your food choices. Only you have the power—moment to moment—to make a balanced lifestyle your highest priority. There is no habit in relation to eating that is more powerful than you are. There is no habit at all that is more powerful that you are. Food is much more than calories, fats, and proteins. Health is so much more than exercise. Happiness is the ever-elusive elixir of life that you have always been chasing, although you never really believed you deserved it. In your relationship to food, you will discover exactly how much you value your existence. You will see clearly exactly how much you are willing to allow nourishment, rejuvenation, and celebration into your deepest sense of self. You are a powerful being, a conscious creator in your life. By taking responsibility for your relationship with food, you reclaim a direct experience of your personal power in the present moment.

The Ashtanga Yoga method starts by asking you to begin the process of self-discovery and inner awareness. It is from this newly enlightened perspective that you can truly know who you are in terms of your relationship with food. Jois always taught that Yoga is self-knowledge. Along the way to the true understanding of the inner self it is not possible merely to adopt dietary guidelines from outside without the ability to understand and feel who you really are. Only once there is a solid basis in self-knowledge can the student even begin to usefully integrate Yogic dietary guidelines. Jois often advised serious students to study Ayurveda as a method of aligning their bodies with Yogic principles.

All human beings exist between two very powerful forces, the Earth below and the cosmic or solar above. Food is a manifestation of the union of these two energies. Foods range on the spectrum of being closer to Earth or closer to the Sun and also range from close to the source and far away from the source. Heavily processed foods are far away from their source. In the Ayurvedic tradition, eating foods that have been stored for a long time are considered a source of imbalance due to their distance from their original source.

Similarly, there are foods that are more earthy and foods that are more solar. Heavier foods are earthy and include animal products like meat and dairy, but also included in this category are root vegetables that grow under the soil. Lighter foods like salad greens, above-ground-growing vegetables, fruits, and juices are closer to their photosynthetic origins. Foods that are of the Sun, that reach you mostly unprocessed, retain their relationship with the Sun and the solar energy contained therein. Included in these categories are also foods that more easily establish balance and foods that more easily instill imbalance. For example, coffee is a liquid that speeds up the brain and often instills imbalance. Similarly, onions and garlic, though being an earthy food, can sometimes stimulate your mind, traditionally stated in the form of desire and lust for external things.

THE THREE MODES OF NATURE

The Yogic diet is a diet aimed at your highest spiritual realization. This is most commonly understood in the Yoga world as a diet that calms and relaxes you, initially, and then leads to self-discovery and union with the Supreme. In the Ayurvedic tradition, this is called the *sattvic* diet. In the material world, traditional Ayurvedic thought states that the universe is composed of three qualities, *sattva* (purity), *rajas* (passion, change) and *tamas* (darkness, inertia).

Sattvic food is considered the purest food and is most suitable for any serious student of Yoga because it nourishes the body, calming and purifying the mind. These foods are primarily bland, whole vegetarian foods including items such as grains, fresh fruits and vegetables, organic dairy products, legumes, nuts and seeds, and honey and herbal teas. Rather than merely vegetarian, truly *sattvic* food is fresh, organic, whole, and cooked or prepared with love. The second category, called *rajasic*, includes foods that stimulate the body and mind for warfare, fighting, and desire. It was the food associated with the warrior, ruling and merchant class in ancient Indian culture. These foods are aimed at stimulating the physical body. They include hot, bitter, sour, dry, salty, and spicy food, including caffeine, fish, eggs, salt, and chocolate. Fast eating is considered *rajasic*, too. The third category consists of *tamasic* food, wherein the energy of the food is withdrawn. Consumption of these foods decreases one's physical strength, mental awareness, and spiritual peace. These foods include meat, poultry, pork, alcohol, onions, garlic, fermented foods, overprocessed foods, canned foods, stale foods, deep fried foods, and rancid oils. Overeating and eating disorders are considered *tamasic*. It is important to remember too that these dietary guidelines come from a culture, context, and history. Just as with any new information, you must use your own common sense to see how much of the Yogic diet is appropriate for you.

Health and happiness are part and parcel of a total life perspective that includes genuine gratitude for the gift of life. The dynamic power of Ashtanga Yoga demands that one be totally conscious—fully aware of your body when you practice. If you are out of balance, you feel it immediately. As a living being, you already have all the seemingly contradictory aspects of your nature within you, and Yoga helps you make peace with every aspect of your being. The work of creating a healthy relationship with food begins first with accepting who you are and what your basic likes and dislikes are and then working with yourself in a patient, persistent, and kind-hearted manner *as you are*. It is from this deep acceptance that one learns through Yoga how to relate to food.

There are certainly foods that are more conducive to practicing Yoga and meditation on a daily basis. Stuff yourself at an all-you-can-eat buffet—with any kind of food whatsoever—and go to a Yoga class. The result is a teaching in itself. But unfortunately, no food type, on its own, in a vacuum, will take you closer to ultimate self-realization—the goal of Yoga. If there is anything that is clear about the teaching of Ashtanga Yoga it is that the path to *samadhi*, total absorption and enlightenment, is a heroic journey that spans the course of many lifetimes. There is nothing you can eat that will get you there in a flash. But there are certainly choices in food that can ease or facilitate the journey.

Just because some Yoga students eat apples and others eat steak does not automatically make one or the other a better Yogi. Ashtanga Yoga teaches that we are all part of the same world, made of the same inner divine substance, and that we all share the same human-angelic heart. Your diet and your overall state of health are a crucial part in your choice to live a spiritual life. However, the single most important factor in determining your relationship with the divine is your choice to respect yourself, respect the natural world, and stay in constant contact with the ineffable force that unites all of creation. Whether you eat an apple or a steak is not the bottom line. If you are a mean person who eats a vegetarian diet and lives a life far away from the divine while practicing *asana*, you are not really a Yogi in the Ashtanga Yoga tradition. On the other hand, if you are a gentle, forgiving person who practices the full lifelong spiritual path of Ashtanga Yoga while occasionally eating a steak you are closer to the heart of Yoga.

Our intimate relationship with food can create a balance and joy that is a celebration of existence. By passing through the permeable membranes of the digestive system, food crosses over physical boundaries. On a biological level, the molecules of food pass from outside to inside and enter the inner space of the body. Once on the inside, these molecules get distributed throughout the body and actually compose the network of muscles, tissues, fibers, organs, skin, flesh, blood, and bones of our being. Ashtanga Yoga asks you to feel and take responsibility for your body in its entirety. It asks students to truly understand that they are what they eat and that like it or not they have 100 percent of the responsibility for all their choices in food. This acceptance comes with a responsibility to build the body of a Yogi. If Yoga practice is a microcosm of life, and food creates the body, then every choice in our intake of food bears a direct result in Yoga and life.

VEGETARIANISM: A PERSONAL CHOICE

Every day, when students get on their Yoga mats, they make a choice about whether they want to continue the path of self-acceptance and growth or whether they want to give in to the voices of doubt and disbelief.

Yoga is about developing discriminating wisdom to see reality clearly, so a Yoga practitioner must know what food really means in our postmodern twenty-first century world. If you practice Yoga, you simply cannot allow yourself to turn a blissfully ignorant eye to the farming practices that produce the food you eat. You must gradually learn to explore what it is you are actually eating, receiving, and saying yes to.

Again, food defines you and your relationship with society. Think about how much of your day revolves around food and you will see how the choices you make about what you put into your mouth say a lot about who you are as a person. Culture is often defined by food preferences. Within each macro-level culture, a subnetwork of social groups exist as well. Yoga practitioners in a sense are carving out a new niche market of conscious consumerism that affects the production of food in the world. Yes, it is too easy and reductionistic to say that simply because we shop at the organic grocery store and eat at the organic restaurant that we are doing something good for the world. Yet at the same time choices in food are extensions of choices in values, showing our sense of principles and wisdom.

You are responsible for everything you eat, both on a personal level in regard to what it does to your body and on a local, national, and global level for what it does to society, nature, and culture. People should get real about what their dollars are going to support and take a conscious stand for what they believe in. Following a vegetarian diet can be seen as a really a sensible thing to do from a variety of standpoints. Raising animals for slaughter takes a lot of the Earth's resources, resources that actually could feed millions of people around the world. The strain that eating meat puts on the Earth is high. Each time someone eats meat they choose to say yes to the entire meat industry, which is behind the production of their food. When one eats meat, one consumes the entire life and death of the animal.

Although there are arguments on both sides of the coin regarding the health of a vegetarian diet, the crucial thing to understand on the path of Yoga is that the choice to follow a Yogic diet is a moral one. This under-standing stems from the *Yoga Sutras* themselves and is embodied in the principle of *ahimsa*, or nonviolence. One of the fundamental commitments on the spiritual path is in fact *ahimsa*, the resolution not to do harm to other beings. This is a noble proclamation that aims to align our actions with our intentions—to be a force of healing in the world.

However, a heartfelt commitment to refrain from harming others does not mean that we will never feel a negative thought again. Nor does it truthfully mean that we will never perpetrate another violent act. Instead, the vow of nonviolence, especially as undertaken by spiritual seekers, stems from a basic recognition—that we have a choice in how we live our lives. Thus, the Yogic path pledges its allegiance to peace through the ancient vow of *ahimsa*. Naturally, one of the easiest ways that Yoga practitioners can stop harming other beings is to stop eating them. This is the advice Jois gave on a most consistent basis to students, that is, to eat a simple vegetarian diet and not to harm other beings. Yoga means to unify, to yoke, to bring together, and one of the most omnipresent things that Yoga brings together is the unity of inner and outer worlds. It is only possible to heartlessly turn animals into a food product when the consumer is separated from the animal as a sentient being. Ashtanga Yoga demands that its students not just intellectualize their connection to all life forms, but actually feel it from within. After such a powerful realization, the illusion of separation falls away and the decision to follow *ahimsa* in terms of a vegetarian diet naturally arises in due course.

The entire process of Yoga is about cultivating your own inner awareness of your lifestyle and its impact on the world around you. Your basic sense of power is the power to choose what you want to be a part of. Whatever you consume enters through the barrier of your body and will actually compose your physical being. What you choose to eat both creates your body and creates the world around you. Agriculture and meat-production practices leave lasting impacts on the Earth and on the means of production. Whatever you eat has passed through multiple human hands. If you eat an apple, someone has either picked it or worked a machine that's picked it. If you eat meat, someone has killed or worked a machine that's killed the animal that you're eating. If you eat butter, a cow has given you milk and a person made the butter. Additionally, there is an entire delivery system that brings your food to stores where you buy it. Each product you buy is a statement about what's valuable to you.

Buying local and organic may be another way to support the kind of relationship with the Earth that is harmonious, well intended, and respectful. Regional concerns are something to consider as well. For example, when local consumers buy and devour apples grown by local farmers, both consumer and producer are connected as part of the food chain, creating a higher connection to the source, both in a psychological and in a pragmatic sense. The money is kept in the local economy, the body is kept in temporal alignment with the local climate, and the consumer and grower are kept in more personal relation to each other.

Imagine this scenario: a consumer living in New York City shops at a local organic grocery store and buys a certified organic apple grown in Washington state instead of buying a locally grown apple that is not certified organic. The question of which one is really "better" becomes a bit tricky because consuming the local apple might mean more to the consumer if he or she gets to know the grower. After talking, the consumer might even learn that the local apple grower doesn't spray and even grows in accordance with many organic standards but doesn't have the certification. Which then is the "better" choice? Again, the question of responsibility in your awareness is up to you.

Every apple seed is unique, just like every human embryo, and the generation of apples requires an understanding of genetics similar to those at play in human reproduction. An apple orchard, whether organic or conventional, uses semi-artificial reproduction because apple seeds are extreme heterozygotes, meaning that each seed contains different material to its parent plants, at least on a genetic level. The slight variation in DNA within the apple is akin to the variation within a human family cluster, primarily producing siblings and occasionally twins.

Doyle and Thyra Fleming run the 170-acre Little Owl Orchard along the Okanogan River and specialize in finding just the right organic alternative to overcultivation of monoculture orchards. They grow three types of cherries, four types of pears, two types of apricots, and five types of apples. They also have a personal breeding ground where roughly 4,000 apple varieties grow free from grafting and budding restrictions. Like a random sample of any population, the fruits range in size from coconut to plum, in shape from spherical to elliptical, in skin from tough to delicate, in smell from watermelon to apple pie, and in taste from banana to spice. Labor is also treated much better on small farms due to the direct relationship between growers and pickers. Even though the income gap still spans a relatively wide margin, the quality of life on small farms is much better for pickers. For example, the Flemings and other local Washington state orchardists often provide long-term housing and other support groups for their pickers so that they can permanently relocate if they so desire. While organic farming is not a panacea for the plight of migrant workers, the steps taken to include the pickers in the farming community are worthy examples of the epistemological differences between conventional and organic agriculture. When you purchase organic apples, you play a vital part in helping create a place for small orchards in the world. The more that you know about agriculture, the source of your food, and the impact of food production, the more your consciousness naturally draws you towards taking each choice at the supermarket with social and environmental responsibility.

Organic agriculture represents a kind of alternative epistemology that you can support every time you go to the supermarket. You must know what you're eating, where's it's coming from and why you're buying it. We are past the age of ignorance, being fully enmeshed in the Information Age where all the answers to your questions are a Google search away. Bring your intelligence and your consciousness into your food choice because every dollar you spend is a way to cast a vote for what you believe in.

It is no accident that the story of our beginning on Earth in the Christian creation myth literally stems from the apple. It is the fabled forbidden fruit whose juices Adam and Eve shared before they were expelled from the proverbial garden. Slice it vertically and you'll see a rendition of female genitalia; slice it horizontally and you'll reveal the five points of a pentagram. An apple a day, keeps the doctor a way. Apple pie is as popularly American as Denny's and McDonald's. More so. I'm writing this essay on a computer called an Apple. There is, of course, the infamous city known as the Big Apple. Notice both the icons of Macintosh and New York City are not just apples, but ones with bites taken from them. Apple nectar contains the juice of human identity; it is our fall from grace, our health and longevity, our nature and culture, our death and resurgence. Perhaps the apple remains with us now because we have never really fallen anywhere other than into ourselves.

While what you put into your body is not who you are, just as what clothes you wear or what job you take is not the essential nature of your being, the food you eat is a kind of extension of your being in the world. Choices in food both reflect the socio-political structures that you support with your grocery money and bring the building blocks of your physical body into being. What you eat gives your body the stuff it needs to make your muscles, joints, bones, blood, organs, brain, hormones, and everything else inside your skin. When food passes through the permeable membrane of your intestines, your mouth or your stomach, you become what you eat in a purely physical sense. The molecules of the food are taken in and begin to percolate throughout your system. So while your spirit and being itself is not composed of this hard, dense, physical matter, your body, earthy in origin, is heavily influenced by what you eat. Your spirit is influenced by your food choices when in the body.

As you take into account just how much there is to be conscious about in your food choices, remember not to lose sight of the larger perspective of the Yoga lifestyle. The idea is to live a happier, healthier life and to be a better person. The choice to be or not to be vegetarian must fit into a larger understanding about the kind of person you want to be every day of your life. The power of your choice in food is not about the food. It is about your state of mind and the balance or imbalance of your perspective and approach to being. Your food choices should never leave you feeling alone in the world. Find a way to both maintain your choice to live a spiritual life and yet go home to your family's house with a smile, an acceptance, and an ability to enjoy holiday dinners with or without the meat. You have to remove the sense of separation and the proclamation about right and wrong out of our gastronomical dialogue. Ashtanga Yoga aims to teach balance, not division. If there is a voice in the practitioner's head that delineates the world into good and bad based on dietary choices, then the whole healing path of Yoga has backfired.

CONCLUSION: THE IMPORTANCE OF BALANCE

It has never been the heart of the spiritual pursuit to sit on a high horse and to pontificate to others. You lose your relationship to others when you judge their choices as being less worthy than yours. When you separate your life from the lives of others, saying that what you do is right and what they do is wrong, you set up harsh divisive lines that are akin to a personal war. This is not the point, nor has it ever been the point, of living a spiritual life.

Jois's most profound teaching is the example he lived in every moment of his life. If being healthy and vegetarian really is the best thing for inner peace, then what his students felt emanating from him was connected to his food choices. The feeling of peace around his being was like an aura of kindness and gratitude. It was not the food that gave him this aura, though he ate and recommended the vegetarian diet that is almost standard in Indian spiritual circles. It is something else that was carried through and the food is merely an expression and an extension of that inner world.

Naturally, food choices change as you become more sensitive to your body and can perceive what is more appropriate for your well-being and spiritual path. Your awareness of the subtle energies of life that flow through you refines your choices in food. Naturally, you want to move away from foods that cause other beings harm; naturally, you want your food to be healthy and support your lifestyle. Key here is that the motivation be natural, not forced or obsessive. If you move into a state of mind that uses your choices in food to create harsh delineations between you and the world, then you have embraced a state and way of being whose harshness and rigidity is far more toxic than any physical substance you can ingest.

Health, in a word, is balance, and Yoga teaches the body and mind to regain their natural state of balance, too. Health is a dynamic equilibrium that holds food, bodily function, emotions, thoughts, physicality, work, love, relationships, and fun in a teetering sphere. By learning how to keep the mind and body unified in challenging Yoga postures, the underlying notion of balance takes root. As students learn to stabilize their Yoga postures, they have to learn to approach their body in a new way. It is through this new way of movement that life changes begin to happen. When students learn to treat their bodies differently in Yoga, they also learn to treat their bodies differently outside of the Yoga room—in day-to-day life.

Ashtanga Yoga inspires its practitioners to move out of an ignorant view of food into an enlightened way of eating. But Yoga itself is no magic solution. Yoga manifests as life transformation if students are willing to apply the lessons learned on the mat to their everyday experience in the world. The most balanced way that Ashtanga Yoga teaches students to understand food is from the perspective of creating a complete lifestyle. If students feel happier eating organic, vegetarian foods as part of their total commitment to balance, health and happiness, then the perfection of Yoga is already achieved.

5

We Are What We Eat: Sri Swami Satchidananda on Vegetarianism

Rev. Sandra Kumari de Sachy

Renowned Yoga master and founder of Integral Yoga International, proponent of interfaith harmony, tireless advocate for world peace, official Citizen of the World, and spiritual guide to thousands of devotees all over the world, Sri Swami Satchidananda, called Gurudev by his disciples, was a lifelong vegetarian.

Born in the South Indian state of Tamil Nadu, in the little village of Chettipalayam, Gurudev grew up in a pious Hindu family.[1] Like most Hindu families in the region, his family followed a strict vegetarian diet. Indeed, most major Hindu sects view vegetarianism as the ideal dietary regimen for human beings. In South India generally and in the state of Tamil Nadu particularly, vegetarianism predominates. Hindus there follow a lifestyle grounded in a religious philosophy that promotes nonviolence, or *ahimsa*, in Sanskrit. Moreover, their tradition holds that eating the flesh of animals is detrimental to one's physical health.

For Western vegetarians, this region is—or at least was—a veritable culinary paradise. In 1995, when my husband and I visited Tamil Nadu, almost every restaurant was completely vegetarian (the very few exceptions posted small signs on the bottom of their windows that said, "Meat served here"). What a treat. In every restaurant we visited, we could order anything listed on the menu. Not surprisingly, though, with the proliferation of television and Internet access and through the influence of Western culture, things aren't what they used to be: I've been told that now many more South Indian restaurants offer meat. In the West, on the other hand, vegetarianism is becoming increasingly popular, and, these days, it's not unusual to find high-quality vegetarian restaurants in most big cities and even in smaller ones. As to the growing popularity of vegetarianism in the United States, I don't think that it would be an overstatement to say that the teachings of Sri Gurudev Swami Satchidananda played a significant role.

YOU ARE WHAT YOU EAT

Today, many Americans probably associate the well-known adage "You are what you eat" with the hippie era of the 1960s, when advocates of natural living and the whole-food diet adopted this dictum to reflect their philosophy of healthy eating. Actually, we can trace the notion and the saying back to eighteenth-century Italy, then to nineteenth century France and Germany, and, more recently, to early twentieth-century America.

In 1728, Bartolomeo Beccari, a distinguished doctor, chemist, and chemistry teacher at Bologna University, decreed, *Quid alius sumus, nisi it unde alimur?* What else are we if not what we eat?[2] Almost a century later, in 1826, the lawyer, judge, and gourmand Jean Anthèlme Brillat-Savarin published a book entitled *Physiologie du Goût, ou Méditations de Gastronomie Transcendante* (*Physiology of Taste, or Meditations of Transcendent Gastronomy*), where he proclaimed: *Dis-moi ce que tu manges, je te dirai ce que tu es.* Tell me what you eat, and I will tell you what you are.[3] Given the reverential, not to say obsessive, attitude that the French exhibit toward food, above all toward their own cuisine, we should not be shocked that Monsieur Brillat-Savarin—who, by the way, was not a vegetarian—was confident enough to assert that he could discern one's essential nature simply by being apprised of one's dietary prerogatives.

Some 40 years later, in 1863/64, the German philosopher/anthropologist and avowed vegetarian Ludwig Andreas Feuerbach wrote an essay entitled "Concerning Spiritualism and Materialism" in which he stated: *Der Mensch ist was er Icht.* The human being is what he eats.[4]

The actual phrase, "You are what you eat," seems to have appeared in English in the 1920s. During that decade, a nutritionist named Victor Lindlahr, who firmly believed that food controlled health, developed a low-carbohydrate diet for weight loss and improved health, which he called the Catabolic Diet. Lindlahr's idea gained some adherents, and the concept appeared in print in a *Bridgeport Telegraph* advertisement for beef: "Ninety per cent of the diseases known to man are caused by cheap foodstuffs. You are what you eat." Later on, in 1942, Lindlahr published *You Are What You Eat: How to Win and Keep Health with Diet.* Though this book introduced the expression "You are what you eat" to the American public, the slogan probably reached a larger audience through radio talks that Lindlahr gave in the 1930s.[5]

A generation later, in the 1960s, the catchy phrase captured a new audience. During this revolutionary era, members of the counterculture grew interested in living a more natural, healthy lifestyle. Their attraction to Eastern teachings and practices introduced them to approaches like Yoga and vegetarianism. These so-called "flower children" of the sixties were searching for ways to liberate themselves from values and conventions that they felt no longer served them. One such seeker was Conrad Rooks. A filmmaker from California, Rooks visited Sri Lanka in 1965 during the time that Gurudev had an ashram (a spiritual community) there.[6]

With its delightful climate and stunning scenery, Sri Lanka was a popular tourist destination, and a number of Western tourists had heard about the young, dynamic Yoga master and his ashram, Satchidananda Thapovanam, in Kandy. So, they came to meet the Swami. And after spending time with Gurudev, they would, invariably, invite him to come to the West. On his part, Gurudev always responded, "Fine. If God wants that, certainly I will do it." Then the tourists would return home, and that would end the matter. That is, until Conrad Rooks appeared.

When Rooks arrived at the ashram to study Yoga with Gurudev, the wheel of fate took a different turn. Planning to settle in for three months, Rooks was soon notified by his office in Paris that he had to return to that city because of some urgent business matter. Reluctantly, he left, and Gurudev didn't hear from him again. About two months later, Gurudev received a round-trip ticket to Paris. The sender was Conrad Rooks. Unable to return to Sri Lanka because he was working on a film (*Chappaqua*), Rooks convinced Gurudev to take some time off to visit him in Europe, and Gurudev left for Paris in March 1966. There, he met Peter Max, who had come from New York to work on the film.[7]

Like Conrad Rooks, Peter Max was captivated by the Swami's blissful demeanor, motivated by his practical teachings, and inspired by his boundless wisdom. Before they parted company, Max told Gurudev straightforwardly: "America needs you." And so it happened that before returning to the ashram in Sri Lanka, Gurudev made a stop in New York, where a number of Max's friends came to meet the charismatic Yogi from India.

Eventually, crowds of hippies came to learn about Yoga from Gurudev. Many of them were stoned on drugs, dirty, and less than respectful when they came to see him. Some of the more conservative students were deeply disturbed by the attitude and appearance of the hippies, imploring Gurudev to turn them away. But he recognized the spiritual yearning and the sincerity in the hearts of these young seekers. Patiently and lovingly, he introduced them to a healthy, balanced lifestyle. He cooked simple Indian vegetarian food for them and then showed them how to do it. He taught them that they could experience peace and joy and the highest states of consciousness through meditation, without the use of hallucinogenic drugs that, at best, offered a temporary high and, at worst, harmed the body and mind.

Soon, a group of people joined together to form an organization based on Gurudev's teachings; they called the organization Integral Yoga, and they founded the Integral Yoga Institute. What was supposed to be a month's vacation for Gurudev turned out to be a year of selfless service, and the "hippies" had become devotees.[8]

When Gurudev finally arrived back in Sri Lanka in February 1967, he found a pile of letters from New York waiting for him. The devotees who sent the letters described the "mass spiritual awakening" that was occurring in the United States, and they urged him to return as soon as possible. Amazingly, even Cecil Lyon, the American ambassador to Sri Lanka, asked him to return to the United States. It seems that Ambassador Lyon had visited the New York Integral Yoga Institute and had seen all the work being done there. He told Gurudev: "Your presence is really needed in America, Swamiji. It would be very nice if you went back."[9] After meditating on the situation for some time, Gurudev realized that he was being guided to return to the United States.

On May 24, 1967, he returned to New York to begin his life in America. Two years later, in the summer of 1969, he was thrust into the spotlight as the swami who was called in to open the Woodstock Festival with a message of peace that would help to create harmony among the hundreds of thousands of mostly young people who had gathered in an upstate New York field, in the rain and mud, for the three-day music festival.

Through the years, students established and continue to establish Integral Yoga centers in the United States and abroad. And until his passing in August 2002, Gurudev traveled nonstop, responding to invitations from all over the world from those who sought his guidance, his wisdom, and his practical application of the ancient Yogic teachings. While some were drawn to the more philosophical and esoteric aspects of Yoga—the law of karma (the law of cause and effect, or action and reaction), the belief in reincarnation, and the attainment of *siddhis* (accomplishments or powers)—everyone seemed to be curious about the effects of food on the body and the mind. Indeed, the topic of diet came up so often in Gurudev's talks that in 1986, his teachings on the subject were published in a book entitled *The Healthy Vegetarian*, which includes a Foreword by cardiologist Dr. Dean Ornish.[10] (Dr. Ornish's bestselling book, *Stress, Diet and Your Heart*, was inspired by Swami Satchidananda's yogic teachings on how to develop and maintain a healthy lifestyle.)

Like Beccari, Brillat-Savarin, Feuerbach, and Lindlahr, Swami Satchidananda ascertained that we are what we eat.[11] Indeed, having attended his weekly *satsangs* (spiritual gatherings) for almost 30 years, I can verify that Gurudev used this very expression, again and again, when discussing the benefits of vegetarianism. To cite one example, during the *satsang* that was held at Satchidananda Ashram on August 12, 1987, someone asked, "Why do we not eat meat here?" Acknowledging that this was such a big topic that it could be the subject of the entire *satsang*, Gurudev decided to give a basic answer: "We have to develop the *sattvic*, or balanced quality, in our life. That means a balanced quality in our body, in our mind, and, for the welfare of all, in the environment." He explained that the meat diet brings mostly the *rajasic*, or restless quality into our system. The human body, he continued, is not made for meat. Our digestive system is more like that of herbivorous animals like cows, horses, and elephants—creatures that have a calm, balanced nature—than it is like the digestive system of restless carnivorous animals like tigers and lions. Finally, Gurudev stated resolutely: "Clean, natural vegetarian food is very important. *You are what you eat.* Remember that truth."[12]

NOURISHING THE BODY, MIND, AND SPIRIT

People often asked Gurudev whether he had a prescription for a healthy lifestyle. He used to reply that he would never offer a "prescription" for a healthy lifestyle, because what might be good for one person might not be suitable for another. As he put it, "One person's nectar is another person's poison. Constitutions vary; lifestyles vary; so each one has to decide what is best for him or her. But I would generally recommend any diet that would be easily digested, that would give enough nutrition, and that would not deposit toxins into the system."[13] His own personal choice was the vegetarian diet, about which he said:

> I have been a vegetarian all my life. I work day and night. I travel twenty days out of the month. Today, I am in Virginia; tomorrow, I might be in Dallas, Texas; the next day, in London. Almost every day, I am lecturing and meeting people, and with all that, I eat only once a day and only vegetarian food. And when I am not traveling, I do manual work, also. I drive a tractor, operate heavy equipment, and ride a horse. My perspiration is always clean, sometimes sweet-smelling like sandalwood. In fact, I tried going for an entire month without taking a bath, and I never smelled bad. I don't fall sick; I never even get the "common cold" or headaches. At one time, a doctor wanted to test the health of my internal organs. He found that my kidneys and heart were those of a twenty-five year-old. [Gurudev was in his 70s at this time.] My chiropractor says that I have the spine of an eighteen-year-old. I sleep very little, only a few hours a night.[14]

From his study of the Yogic teachings and through his own personal experience, Gurudev had come to know that diet plays a vital role in our physical health. But he had learned, too, that diet plays an equally important part in our mental and spiritual wellbeing. Generally speaking, most people think about food in relation to how it affects the physical body. Yogis, on the other hand, believe that if we want to enjoy optimum health, we need to broaden our awareness by observing that what we eat also influences our mind and, ultimately, our spirit. This holistic approach to diet characterizes Gurudev's teachings on vegetarianism.

THE BODY

Why Vegetarianism?

According to Gurudev, the natural diet for human beings is a vegetarian diet. Categorizing mammals into two major groups, the flesh eating and the vegetarians, he pointed out the following differences to illustrate how human beings belong to the latter group.

Flesh-eating animals have long teeth with which to tear raw animal flesh from bones; they have rough tongues so that they can lick flesh from bones; they have sharp, strong claws to catch and kill their prey; their intestines are only about two to three times the length of their body, which means that meat can pass through their systems quickly before it becomes putrid; and they gulp their food. Conversely, herbivorous animals have intestines that are six or seven times their body length, because their systems don't have to push food through rapidly; they have a different type of pH in their saliva and their stomach; they have digestive enzymes in their saliva; they don't gulp their food but begin digesting while the food is still in their mouth; and they don't have sharp claws or very rough tongues. As for human beings, we also have flat, grinding teeth like vegetarian animals; our intestines are about 26 feet long, six to seven times our body's length; we don't have rough tongues or sharp claws (at least not in the literal sense); and our pH, which contains digestive enzymes, is similar to that of vegetarian animals.[15]

Gurudev believed and taught that we are meant to be vegetarians, that fruits and nuts, vegetables, and grains are intended to be our food. Invariably, someone attending a talk would argue that at least some human beings must be meant to eat meat. What about the Inuits or Tibetans? How would they feel if someone told them that they were meant to be vegetarians and must give up meat? Always an advocate of the common-sense approach, Gurudev would reply that he would never advocate a vegetarian diet in an environment where even grass couldn't grow. In such an environment one must eat animals in order to survive. Nonetheless, in *The Healthy Vegetarian*, he noted: "The average life span of an Eskimo [Inuit] is twenty-seven and a half years. Compare this with the life span of the Hunzas of Pakistan, whose diet is primarily vegetarian. Recorded ages of 110 are not uncommon among their population."[16]

Gurudev's approach was clear: if we live in an environment where we can get the type of food that most suits our nature, that is, vegetarian food, we should certainly do so. He asserted that a diet of fruit, vegetables, grains, legumes, nuts and milk products (provided, of course, that one isn't allergic to any of these foods) is the best diet for promoting good health, because it doesn't cram our systems with lots of toxins in the way that animal matter does. When an animal is killed, its corpse quickly begins to decay. When we eat the flesh, we're eating dead matter. It's different with vegetables. Vegetables dehydrate, yes, but it takes a long time for them to decay. To illustrate this point, Gurudev used to say that if you eat half of a vegetable, you can plant the other half and that half will grow again, because it's still a living organism. He used spinach as an example, maintaining that if you cut the stem of a spinach plant into 10 parts and eat the leaves but plant the stem, eventually, you will get 10 new spinach plants. "Can you do that with a lamb?" he would ask. "Can you eat its leg and then make the other parts grow into another lamb?"[17]

As to the toxicity of meat, Gurudev insisted that even if a veterinarian certified an animal as healthy before the animal was slaughtered, the adrenalin that courses through its body—just as it courses through ours when we're frightened or stressed—affects the animal's every cell, imbuing the cells with toxins and hormones. Regrettably, these undesirable toxins and hormones remain in the meat that human beings ingest. And, again, because our intestines are so long, decayed flesh becomes putrid in the body before it can be digested and eliminated, causing toxicity. The toxins that remain in the body become the cholesterol that hardens the arteries, a condition known as atherosclerosis, which can result in high blood pressure, heart attacks, and strokes. What's more, the toxins that are eliminated cause foul perspiration odor. He made the case that "if everyone were to become a vegetarian, we could close all the deodorant factories." In this light, he described the "television commercials in which a young man [or woman] comes up to talk to a young woman [or man] only to have her make a face and run away. So, he goes and sprays something in his mouth, and then all the girls come flocking around him!"[18] Gurudev stated firmly that vegetarians living on pure food have no need to disguise their perspiration odor, because their perspiration can emit a sweet, flowerlike fragrance—jasmine or sandalwood, for example—which others would find quite attractive. Even more graphically, he maintained that the excrement of vegetarians who eat the proper food in the proper quantity will be well formed, will pass out of the body in "softish balls" and will not smell bad unless there is something wrong with the stomach or intestines.[19]

WHAT ABOUT PROTEIN?

Olfactory and scatological issues aside, perhaps the most frequently asked question put to Gurudev—and, perhaps, to all vegetarians—was: how will I get enough protein on a vegetarian diet? He taught that although it's true that meat contains a great deal of protein, the fact is that our systems don't require such rich, concentrated protein. He also pointed out that even meat-eating animals, as well as meat-eating human beings, normally eat only herbivorous rather than carnivorous animals. Our protein, he maintained, should be as close to its natural source as possible, so that an herbivorous animal serves as a better source of protein than does a carnivorous one. But, he asserted, eating vegetables themselves provides us with the best source of protein. And beans, lentils, avocados, and dairy products also provide protein that is easy for us to digest.

Dairy? Eggs?

Gurudev taught that dairy products don't have the concentrated fat that meat has and that milk, a whole food, is very *sattvic*, that is, conducive to a peaceful mind. On the other hand, he also said that too much dairy causes mucus and phlegm, especially if one is lactose intolerant (the inability to digest dairy because of the lack of the enzyme lactose, a component of milk and other dairy products).

It's important to note, too, that while Gurudev described dairy products as *sattvic*, or balanced, his point of reference was South India, where he grew up. Cows there are worshipped, revered as sacred beings; they roam freely, eat organically, and are not contaminated by the hormones and antibiotics that are given to cattle raised like commodities on the strictly-for-profit factory farms that provide most of the dairy produced in the United States. Moreover, because of the tropical climate, cow's milk in India does not contain the large amount of fat that we find in milk produced in the United States; cow's milk in India is thinner and more nutritious, because there is much less fat. Still, Gurudev contended, milk is not healthy for us to consume, especially in the West where the high fat content of milk makes it difficult to digest, resulting in increased cholesterol levels and even rheumatic and arthritic conditions.

Another vital consideration for vegetarians is that it is standard practice in the U.S. dairy industry to either slaughter male calves born to dairy cows or to sell them to the beef industry to be slaughtered. Many vegetarians find this disturbing, feeling that by eating dairy, they are contributing to the suffering of the animals. During a talk on June 9, 1990, Gurudev responded to this concern: "Yes, it's true. Indirectly, you are contributing to this situation. . . . This is one of the reasons why we don't keep [dairy cows] at Yogaville."[20] He conceded that some people feel that they need dairy in their diet because it provides more protein than vegetables and grains, He recommended that in this case, one should limit the use of dairy products, including fat-free milk. He held that, strictly speaking, adults don't need milk; after all, it's only adult humans who drink milk. "Certainly," he wrote in *The Healthy Vegetarian*, "we can live very well without milk products, eating only fruits, vegetables, legumes, grains, and nuts." Alternatively, he counseled that if you do use milk products, at least offer a prayer or a blessing to the animal that gave you its milk.

When asked whether eggs were suitable to a vegetarian diet, Gurudev responded that eggs, even unfertilized eggs, "partake of the same quality as flesh." To illustrate this point, he said that when you break an egg and leave it, the egg very quickly begins to decay, and it emits a foul odor just as meat does.[21] Needless to say, eggs are not part of the Yogic diet.

To Eat Raw or Cooked Food? That Is the Question

These days, more and more vegetarians are converting to a raw food diet. When asked for his opinion on whether a raw food or cooked food diet is the best approach to vegetarianism, Gurudev replied:

Food eaten whole and raw has a lot of bulk. For example, when you eat a whole raw apple, you get bulk from the cellulose coating. Almost everything should be eaten with the husk on it—vegetables, fruits, beans, and even grains. We spend money to take the bran out of the wheat for white flour products; then we spend money to buy extra bran to supplement our diet. If we eat products in their whole state, we will get plenty of bulk.

There is yet another advantage to eating raw food. We consume much less of the same food when it is not cooked. Take cauliflower. The average person could not eat even half of a raw cauliflower. But if it were cooked, the same person could easily eat the entire vegetable. By eating uncooked food, we save food, we get more bulk, and, at the same time, we save time and energy in preparing it. I often say that the day human beings learned to cook their food was the day they began laying the foundations for the hospitals.[22]

Once, a student wondered how a vegan diet without dairy products could provide enough vitamin B-12. Addressing this concern, Gurudev stated that if we eat plain raw vegetables and chew them very well and then digest them well, the body, a veritable chemical factory, has the capacity to convert one substance (vitamin or mineral, for instance) into 10 others. To illustrate this marvel, he explained that a cow eats only grass, yet the milk that it gives is filled with vitamins that were converted from the grass. In the same way, he maintained, our body can create whatever it needs out of one food. As far as Gurudev was concerned, the preoccupation with certain kinds of diet was a modern phenomenon bordering on obsession.

According to him, it wouldn't matter if we ate one diet all through our lifetime. Again, he used the cow as an example. A cow eats the same food throughout its life, converting the grass into many vitamins. We can do the same thing, provided we eat well, chew well, digest well, and assimilate well. However, Gurudev did affirm that for optimum digestion, assimilation, and good health, first and foremost is that we eat only when we're really hungry. He supported this principle with a quote from a South Indian scripture, the *Tirukkural*, which says: [The] body never needs medicines or even vitamins if only you eat after you know full well that you have completely digested what you ate before.[23]

At the same time, Gurudev's approach to any subject was never one-dimensional. Though he did say that "the day human beings started cooking their food, they began laying the foundations for hospitals and clinics"[24] and taught that fruits, roots, vegetables, nuts, and so on were our natural foods, at the same time, he did not advocate that we all revert to a raw food diet. Recognizing that we have been removed from such a diet for so long that our digestive systems have become accustomed to eating cooked food, he recommended steaming as the best alternative to eating raw food. And if steamed food is not an option, then the second-best alternative is gently cooked food, including vegetables.[25]

Sugar = Satan?

Once, during one of Gurudev's talks, someone brought up the issue of sugar. Aware that too much sugar in the diet weakens the immune system and causes poor health, the questioner inquired dramatically, "Is sugar Satan?" In no uncertain terms—and to some listeners' delight—Gurudev replied: "Don't say that sugar is Satan. Sugar comes from God."

However, he didn't stop there. He went on to say that if we eat sugar within limits, it tastes good; but if we eat sugar in excess, eventually, it won't taste so good, and we won't like it any more. He also said that while the refined white sugar that we normally eat is not good for us, it's alright to eat natural sugar, provided we eat it in moderation. Having worked for a time in a sugar factory, he had first-hand knowledge of sugar processing.

He described how companies spend a lot of money to extract the molasses from sugar and how they use bleach to make the sugar white. In contrast, natural sugar (called jaggery in India), contains a great deal of molasses, which is good for the health. He cautioned, though, that even natural sugar, like every other food, should be eaten within limits. God, he stated, never made anything bad; instead, we make it bad by overdoing it. He concluded his answer with a saying translated from the South Indian Tamil language: "If it goes beyond the limit, even nectar becomes poison." In other words, he added, "Everything within limits is okay."[26]

The Mono-Diet

The mono-diet, which refers to eating only one food item by itself for some time rather than putting several different foods into the stomach at the same time, is often used in the naturopathic approach to healing. Gurudev encouraged his students to go on a mono-diet from time to time, because when you eat just one type of fruit, vegetable, or grain, your body digests the food more easily and assimilates it better. When it comes to fruit, he advised that if one piece of fruit, say an apple, doesn't satiate your hunger, you can eat more, even up to four apples. If you decide to eat carrots, eat only carrots for your meal. As Gurudev put it, "Your stomach will be grateful to you, because it will have just one thing to do; digestion will be much quicker and easier."[27] Why? Because each food requires a different amount of time to digest and utilizes different enzymes.

Food Combining

Again, though, Gurudev's perspective was broad. For those who felt that they needed a little more variety, he suggested eating two or three foods together, making sure, however, that the particular foods would be digested in a similar manner and in the same amount of time. Take the combination of raw and cooked food as an example. To ensure good digestion, it's really helpful *not* to eat raw and cooked food at the same meal, as they're broken down differently in the body.

Additionally, if you're eating solid foods, stick to solids; conversely, if you're eating liquids or drinking, have only liquids. This idea, Gurudev conceded, is practically unknown in the West, where people usually drink with their meals or end a meal with a beverage. He said that even water shouldn't be taken during a meal of solid food, because it will dilute the digestive juices. According to the yogic diet, liquids should be taken an hour or two after solid food. Gurudev explained that if we do get thirsty while eating, it means that we're not chewing our food enough before swallowing it.[28] He often reminded us that we should drink our solids and eat our liquids. More explicitly, when we're eating, we should chew the food well until the solids break down and become liquid, mixing completely with our saliva. And when we're drinking, we should mix the liquid well in our mouth and swallow it slowly as we do when we chew.

Gurudev also pointed out another bad habit that many people have: they drink milk with other foods. Milk, he said, is a whole food in itself and should be taken alone, although if you really feel that you have to have something with it, you could have a banana. Citrus should never be taken at the same time as milk. While this may seem like common sense—who would think of pouring orange juice into a glass of milk?—it is common, at least in the United States, for people to have a glass of orange juice and a bowl of cereal with milk for breakfast.

A final word about food combining. Dinned into my consciousness is a little limerick that Gurudev taught us about eating melon (which digests rather quickly): *Eat it alone, or leave it alone!*

What to Eat

In discussions about what to eat and how much to eat, Gurudev encouraged his students to eat a plain and simple diet, making it clear to us that we don't need as much food as we often think we do. Referring to his own diet, he would say that because his mind is always relaxed and never stressed, his body doesn't need much food. As he worded it, "My fuel economy is very good." He explained that people waste a lot of energy in worrying, that anxiety about the future drains a great deal of their energy. Figuratively speaking, people who worry "drain their batteries completely." As a result, these people have to eat more to regain energy. Gurudev never drained his vital energy, his *prana*, so he could live on very little. He revealed, in fact, that he could even live on air alone. In the late 1940s, he lived for several months on three cups of milk a day and nothing else during a time when he was working hard at the ashram where he lived.[29]

Gurudev was able to live this way and to sustain good health because he wasn't wasting his energy. He claimed, in fact, that if we don't waste our energy, we can even *gain* energy directly from the elements. He explained that through food, we obtain the elements, but if we know how to take energy directly from the elements, then we don't need any food at all. He remarked that people who live in Western countries often fall sick because they overeat, recalling that during World War II, when there were food shortages in most European countries, many hospitals in those countries were empty because people weren't falling sick from overeating.

According to Gurudev, we have to understand our own systems. We have to ask ourselves, How much energy have we used up during our activities and how much food do we need to replace this energy? To find the answers, we need to ask our stomach whether it really needs more food, whether it used up what it took in earlier. And unless the stomach—not the mind—answers that it's ready for more food, we should not eat. As he astutely put it, most people eat for the two *t*'s, that is, for the *tongue* and the *time*. Instead, he insisted, we should eat for the third *t*: for the *tummy*.

To underscore this point, he would quote the great Indian saint Thiruvalluvar, who said: "The body will never need medicine if food is never taken without making sure that the stomach has digested what was given to it before."[30] His point, of course, is that hunger is the only dependable clock and the only reliable sign that can tell you when to eat. Just as importantly, however, we need to be able to recognize true hunger. Gurudev used to say that if our hunger "pangs" go away within a short time, then what we felt was not true hunger. Such pangs, he explained, are grounded in habitual eating patterns that create a false sense of hunger, and they vanish in about a half hour. True hunger pangs, on the other hand, won't go away until we eat something.

Additionally, when talking about when and what to eat, Gurudev recommended that breakfast should be a light meal, fruit or cereal, for example. This line of reasoning surprises many Americans when they encounter the yogic approach to diet, because they are taught from a young age that it's important to begin the day with a hearty breakfast—the "breakfast of champions" approach. But from the yogic perspective, when we first wake up, our digestive fire is not very strong; it's still partly asleep, so our morning meal should be light. Lunch, however, can be a heavier meal, since we have plenty of time to digest; also, we'll be using the energy from that food later on in the day. Supper, like breakfast, should be light, and we should finish the evening meal at least two hours before going to sleep. If we go to bed with undigested food in the stomach, some of the energy will be used to digest and we won't get a very good rest.

Speaking about digestion, Gurudev held that taking time for digestion is very important. He told us that in India there is a saying: "When the stomach is full, the brain is dull."[31]

Of course, at one time or another, we've probably all experienced the yawning and the sluggish feeling that come after eating a heavy meal. When we're filled up with heavy food, we're not able to think well, because the blood circulation that normally goes to the brain has gone down to the stomach. And if we force the blood to go up to the brain, for instance, if we go back to work right after eating a heavy meal, our stomach will suffer. So if our job doesn't allow us time to rest after lunch, then we need to eat a lighter lunch and an earlier dinner.

With respect to what we should eat, Gurudev stressed the importance of taking into consideration the activities in which we are engaged, a notion, he said, that goes almost unrecognized in Western societies. He stated that the proportion of solids and liquids in our diet should go hand in hand with the type of work that we do. In *The Healthy Vegetarian* he wrote,

> The more physical labor that you do, the more solid food you should take. If you do more mental work, you can take more liquid food and not so much solid food. A person doing hard manual labor might need three meals of solid food a day; whereas a desk worker, who is mostly sitting and thinking, should not eat more than one solid meal a day to keep in good health. People who are mostly meditating or doing things with complete ease can take more energy from the air itself. From solid, to liquid, to gas: if the need is for physical energy, we take food from a solid source; if the need is mental, from liquid; and if the need is spiritual, then from a gaseous source. Children who are growing need quite a lot of physical energy to make their bodies grow well, so they can eat solid food quite often. (p. 31)

In general, Gurudev's basic guidelines for a diet that will keep us healthy are

- a diet that is plain and simple;
- a diet that will keep the mind calm and the body relaxed and toxin free;
- a diet that agrees with the body's system;
- a diet that is easy to digest;
- a diet that is economical;
- a diet that requires a minimum amount of time to prepare;
- a diet that is easy to clean up after eating.

To sum up, I offer one of Gurudev's favorite Indian sayings: If you eat once a day, you are a *Yogi* (a well-balanced, spiritual person); if you eat twice a day, you are a *Bhogi* (someone who enjoys the world); and if you eat three times a day, you are a *Rogi* (*roga* means sickness in Sanskrit). From his perspective as a Yogi and, again, from his own life experience, Gurudev observed that if we eat three times a day, we will probably fall sick pretty often.

How to Eat

Presumably, most of us think quite a bit about *what to eat* and *when to eat*. I wonder, though, how many of us think about *how to eat*. Fortunately, Gurudev offered instruction along these lines, too. He taught that how we eat our food is an essential component of good health.[32]

First of all, he noted, digestion actually begins in the mouth, where the saliva contains digestive enzymes. Therefore, we should be using all of our 32 teeth to chew, and we should use them to chew well, really well. Then, he recommended that we make sure to eat when our body and mind are relaxed; it's always best not to eat when we're upset, angry, or agitated, because, as he put it, we will be—literally—poisoning our stomach. Furthermore, it's also better not to prepare food for anyone else when we're upset, because the negative vibrations emanating from us will be absorbed into the food that we're cooking, affecting those who eat it. That's why it's best to prepare food when our mind is calm.

Gurudev also recommended sitting silently for a few minutes before we begin to eat, consciously taking time to relax the body and to let go of any disturbing or distracting thoughts. Saying a short prayer of gratitude before the meal is also beneficial. Even further, he advised us to take our meals in silence. In silence, we can concentrate on the food while we're eating it, which means that we will digest it better and, as a result, enjoy it more. How often do we get so engrossed in conversation while we're eating that we don't even really taste the food? Then again, if we are socializing and there is conversation during a meal, at least it should be light and pleasant. As far as Gurudev was concerned, "A 'business' lunch or dinner does not do justice either to the business or to the meal. The business deal will be sounder if our mind is only on the business and if part of our energy is not going into digestion. And our stomach will be happier if we focus all our attention on our food while we're eating." Besides, this kind of mindfulness during meals will help us eat less if we tend to eat more food than we need.

Fasting

According to Gurudev, fasting is a natural process, and it is practiced in many spiritual traditions. Even animals fast.

When he talked about fasting, Gurudev described the body as a factory. In a factory, the machines work all week; then, they're given some down time so that they can be cleaned and overhauled and, also, so that they can take a rest. Similarly, the body's digestive system needs a little break from its ordinary routine in order to function well—even when we've been eating the right food. This down-time allows the body to eliminate any toxins or burn excess fat that we might have put into it. As Gurudev articulated it, the body "overhauls itself and gets ready for the next day's work." Actually, if you eat the proper foods and have only a light supper in the evening, your system enjoys a mini-fast every night. During this time, it gets cleaned and the stomach gets some rest. Unfortunately, though, our heavy suppers and late evening meals and snacks often prevent this respite and cleansing process. Hence, according to the Yogic teachings, longer fasts of one day or more are advisable.

For a healthy person with a good diet, Gurudev recommended one day of fasting a week, from after dinner through the entire next day and night, ending the fast with a light breakfast, perhaps fruit or a little yoghurt and cucumber. He avowed that such a fasting routine would take care of small problems in the body before they could become big problems. For those who have a great deal of toxic material in the body, it might take from 2 to 10 days to eliminate the toxins.

So, how will you know when to end a fast? There are definite signs: you'll feel light; your saliva will be clean, clear, and sweet tasting; your tongue will no longer be coated; your vision will be sharper; all your senses will be keener; you won't feel dull or drowsy; you'll experience an amazing feeling of strength, not necessarily to do strenuous physical work but to run as though to fly.

Further, Gurudev maintained that if fasting brings so many benefits to healthy people, it's particularly important for weak or ill people to fast, because when your body is sick, your stomach is also sick, and when you eat, your sick stomach has to work even harder to digest. Instead, it's wiser to allow the stomach to rest and heal. To highlight this teaching, he would quote a well-known maxim, popular among Hindus of his day: "Fasting is the best medicine."

Actually, when you're ill, you often don't feel like eating anything anyway. It's a natural reaction. In this respect, Gurudev said that to help cure almost any ailment, you should stay away from food until your symptoms subside and you feel hungry. For when you give your system a rest, your vital energy acts as an "inner doctor," burning up and eliminating the toxins that created the ailment.

To reiterate, when you fast, you eliminate toxins from the system, digest the undigested food, assimilate any extra fat stored in the body, and, thus, return to normal health.

In his experience, Gurudev found that the best way to fast is simply to drink plain water, especially if you're fasting for health reasons (on certain religious holidays, some people don't even take water during a fast). However, if you find that too difficult, you can fast on fruit juice diluted with water. Hearing that some people fast on carrot juice, drinking four or five glass a day, with each glass containing the juice of six or seven carrots (you might be consuming 30 or 40 raw carrots a day), he advised against this practice. Rather, he recommended fruit juices like grape or orange, juices that are more watery. He highly recommended watermelon juice for fasting.

Another of Gurudev's recommendations vis-à-vis fasting is the use of enemas and purgatives. He said that taking an enema once or even twice a day while fasting is very good for the system. Since the system (including the colon) gets heated during a fast, with moisture from the waste matter being absorbed back into the system, it's important to eliminate the waste. He also suggested taking a purgative—he recommended castor oil—to clean the bowels before beginning the fast. Cleaning the bowels first, he said, is particularly important if you're fasting in order to cure an infection, because any inflammation in the body and any swelling become more painful if the stomach or colon are still heavy with undigested, fermented matter.

Sometimes when you fast, you may experience some unpleasant symptoms, because toxins are being removed from the organs, glands, and tissues into the bloodstream and are then being eliminated through perspiration, breath, urine, and solid waste. You may get a headache, for instance; if so, drink more water. Or you may feel nauseated; in this case, drink lots of water and then throw it up. At times, you may feel weak, as though you've lost all your strength. This is fine. However, if this sensation does occur, don't do anything strenuous for a while, but continue your fast. Additionally, your tongue will get coated, and your breath and saliva may small bad, all signs that toxins are being released and eliminated.

Gurudev also advocated sunbathing, when possible, during fasting, because you'll perspire and cleanse even more; sunbathing, he said, is like a very mild sauna that doesn't stress the system. Nasal cleansing and stomach-washing techniques are also beneficial. These methods are called *kriyas* in Sanskrit. (For more information about *kriyas*, consult *Integral Yoga Hatha*, by Yogiraj Sri Swami Satchidananda, 3rd edition. Integral Yoga Publications, Buckingham, 1995.)

Finally, while we normally associate fasting with the body, Gurudev made us aware of the higher significance of this practice. Fasting, he taught, helps to calm the mind. For when you gain mastery over the senses—in this case, the tongue—indirectly, you gain mastery over the mind. Thus, if you aspire to gain control over your mind, fasting can help you to reach the goal. And this, he told us, is one of the reasons why fasting is so often associated with spiritual and religious observances.[33]

THE MIND

The Three *Gunas*

To fully understand Gurudev's teachings on the relationship between diet and the mind—specifically, the psychological benefits of a vegetarian diet—it's important to know something about the three *gunas*, or the

qualities of nature. The philosophy behind the concept of the *gunas* is set
forth in Book I, *sutra* 16, of Patanjali's *Yoga Sutras*: *Tat Param Purusa
Khyater Gunavaitrsnyam*. In English, "When there is non-thirst for even
the *gunas* (constituents of nature) due to realization of the *Purusha* (true
Self), that is supreme non-attachment."[34]

In his commentary on the *Yoga Sutras*, Gurudev writes that, originally,
the world, or *Prakriti* in Sanskrit, was *avyakta*, unmanifested. When *Prakriti*
began to manifest, the ego came first; then, individuality emerged; and,
finally, the mind materialized. From the mind, the *tanmatras* (a term that
signifies the essence of all objects) appeared, followed by the gross elements. This, from the Yogic standpoint, is our natural evolution. This is
why, according to Yoga, God didn't create anything. Yoga says that God is
pure consciousness and *Prakriti*, the world, is there, too, its nature being
to evolve and then to dissolve. *Prakriti*, in its unmanifested state, has both
matter and force. When nature is in an unmanifested condition, the force
is static or dormant. This force, or *prana*, has three components called the
gunas: *rajas*, *tamas*, and *sattva*, or the active state, the passive state, and the
tranquil state, respectively. When all three of these qualities are in equilibrium, they don't affect matter. But even a little disturbance in the *gunas*
creates motion in matter, giving rise to all the various forms; and that is
how the entire universe, with all its elements, appears. We can observe
the *gunas* at work—and at play—in our personalities and even in the food
that we eat. That is to say, some people are very active, even restless;
others are slow and sluggish; and there are those who are tranquil and
composed. In fact, in one of the principal scriptures of Yoga, the *Bhagavad
Gita*, Lord Krishna offers a lengthy discourse on the various temperaments
and the types of foods that attract them.[35]

First, he describes calm people and their preferred diet:

> Those of tranquil temperament [*sattvic*] prefer foods that increase vitality,
> longevity and strength; foods that enhance physical health and make the
> mind pure and cheerful; foods with substance and natural flavor; foods that
> are fresh, with natural oils and agreeable to the body. (17:8)

In his commentary, Gurudev explains that Krishna describes for us the
nature of *sattvic* foods: they enhance vitality, vigor, energy, good health,
and joyfulness; they are tasty and fresh, with a little oil (sesame and sun-
flower seeds, for example), and easy to digest. Such foods as fruit, nuts,
milk products, vegetables (raw and cooked), cooked grains, peas and beans
are considered to be *sattvic*. However, when they're mixed with lots of
spices and become hot or sour, they are considered to be *rajasic*. Gurudev
adds: "And these foods should not only be healthy and energizing; even

just seeing the plate of food should cheer you. The food shouldn't just be thrown on the plate in a big mess."[36]

Then, Krishna talks about restive people and their favorite foods:

> Those of a restless, compulsive temperament [*rajasic*] prefer foods that are very spicy or very sour, piping hot, bitter-dry, or quite salty. Such foods give rise to discomfort, pain and disease and, therefore, dismay. (17:9)

Referring to Krishna's comments about the deleterious effects of *rajasic* foods, Gurudev stressed that it isn't necessary to eat extremely spicy, hot food. He reminded us that just because Yoga comes from India, it doesn't mean that if we practice Yoga, we need to copy everything that's done in India. As a matter of fact, he said, eating hot food even once in a while isn't that good for us, because as much as a day or two after eating very spicy food, we may feel our entire alimentary canal burning. And from a more subtle perspective, Yoga teaches that if we're practicing meditation, it is best to refrain from eating spicy foods, including garlic and onions, because these foods agitate the mind, making it difficult for us to meditate. In addition, those who practice celibacy would be wise to forego such stimulants as garlic and onions.

So how do we know when food is *rajasic*? As Gurudev depicted it, "If your tongue tingles and burns, or the eyes get bloodshot and teary, or the nose runs and the stomach burns, know that you are eating *rajasic* food."[37] Not a pretty picture!

On the other hand, when used properly, some spices can be utilized medicinally. Gurudev recommended *rasam*, a very peppery soup that South Indians take when they have a cold, because black pepper can help to control cold symptoms. He told us that for stomach problems or for worms in the stomach, South Indian mothers add more turmeric to their dishes, because turmeric is a good antiseptic. To treat inflammations, they add something sour. We can use food, he said, as medicine; but medicine should be taken only as needed, not just because the tongue likes it. And by the way, meat and other flesh are also *rajasic*

Lastly, Krishna describes the lethargic types and their culinary preferences:

> Those of a dull and lazy temperament [*tamasic*] choose foods that are stale and tasteless, overcooked or left overnight, spoiled, rotting or even putrid. Such foods have lost their vitality and nutrition. (17:10)

Generally, the *tamasic* category includes foods that are old, overcooked, very cold, or moldy. Regarding the above verse, Gurudev commented that while most of us wouldn't eat stale, rotting food, it seems to be quite a common habit in the United States to eat food that is cooked and kept overnight. He recalled that when he came to America in 1966, a couple invited him to their country home for the weekend. On Sunday afternoon, when they were getting ready to return home, he found the wife in the kitchen preparing a big pot of cooked rice and vegetables. He wondered why she had cooked so much food, since there weren't many people in the group. The woman confided that every weekend, before leaving the countryside, she cooked enough food for the coming week; when she arrived home, she put the food in the refrigerator, and the family warmed some up every night for supper. Gurudev was shocked—this was never done in India. He had learned that even if leftover food looked okay, it was still old food that had lost its freshness and vitality. He also felt that because Americans thought of their country as "the land of plenty," they wasted food. Some people, he noticed, weren't even respectful toward food. The way he saw it, food is an expression of God.[38]

Concerning the relationship between food and the mind, while certain personality types are attracted to particular kinds of food, conversely, these same foods directly affect the personality. For example, in the *Bhagavad Gita*, Lord Krishna tells us that *rajasic* food creates restlessness in the mind. Thus, if our goal is to keep our mind calm and to remain peaceful, as in the practice of Yoga, we wouldn't want to eat a lot of hot, spicy food or use too much garlic and onion. And, we wouldn't eat meat, which makes us active in a restless, sometimes aggressive manner. Likewise, if we wish to remain alert and active, then we should stay away from those heavy, oily, overcooked, mind-numbing *tamasic* foods that make us dull and boring.

Food for Thought

Gurudev taught that the manner in which we eat can also create a body and mind that is *sattvic*, *rajasic*, or *tamasic*. As an example, if we don't chew *sattvic* food well, it will ferment in the body and may result in *tamas*, or lethargy. Also, if we overeat right before going to sleep, we will become *tamasic*.

So, if want to enjoy a balanced mind, a dynamic personality, a healthy body, and a peaceful and productive life, take the advice of the great Yogis, past and present: make your diet a *sattvic* one and eat it in the proper manner. And always remember that diet shapes not only the body, but also the mind and the spirit.

THE SPIRIT

The Yoga of Synthesis

Gurudev called his approach to Yoga "Integral Yoga," that is, the Yoga of synthesis. Integral Yoga takes into consideration all the aspects of the individual—the physical, emotional, mental, intellectual, social, and spiritual—exemplifying the branch of Yoga known as *Raja Yoga*. Although *Raja Yoga* (*raja* is Sanksrit for "royal") is generally thought of as the path of meditation that leads to control of the mind, effectively this branch of Yoga represents an integral approach to life. *Raja Yoga* takes into account the entire life of the individual, its ultimate aim being the "total transformation of a seemingly limited physical, mental, and emotional person into a fully illumined, thoroughly harmonized and perfected being—from an individual with likes and dislikes, pains and pleasures, successes and failures, to a sage of permanent peace, joy, and selfless dedication to the entire creation."[39]

As I noted previously, the principal text of *Raja Yoga* is Patanjali's *Yoga Sutras*. The nearly 200 *sutras*, or threads of meaning, are apportioned into four sections. The first, *Samadhi Pada*, or the Portion on Contemplation, presents the theory of Yoga and a description of the most advanced levels of the practice of *samadhi*, which is translated into English as "contemplation" or the "super-conscious state." The second section, *Sadhana Pada*, the Portion on Practice, offers philosophy of a more practical nature. In this section, Patanjali expounds on the "eight limbs of Yoga." The third section, *Vibhuti Pada*, is the Portion on Accomplishments, and it describes the powers and accomplishments that can be achieved by the dedicated practitioner. The fourth and final section is called *Kaivalya Pada*, the Portion on Absoluteness, which discusses Yoga philosophically from the cosmic perspective.

The section most relevant to Gurudev's teachings on vegetarianism is the second one, the Portion on Practice. In this section, Patanjali lists the eight stages of Yoga practice. He refers to these stages as the "eight limbs," which is why the *Yoga Sutras* are also known as *Ashtanga Yoga*, or Eight-limbed Yoga. He lists these eight stages in the following order:

1. *yama* (abstinence): nonviolence, truthfulness, nonstealing, continence, and nongreed
2. *niyama* (observance): purity, contentment, accepting but not causing pain, study of spiritual books and worship of God or self-surrender
3. *asana* (posture)
4. *pranyama* (breath control)
5. *pratyahara* (sense withdrawal)
6. *dharana* (concentration)
7. *dhyana* (meditation)
8. *samadhi* (contemplation, absorption or superconscious state)

The order of this listing is not arbitrary. Rather, it delineates an intentional, stage-by-stage approach that serves to guide Yoga practitioners in their pursuit of Self-realization. Although each of the eight limbs is equal to the others and each is a necessary practice, notice that the first two limbs are *yama* and *niyama*. Why did Patanjali place them at the top of his list? Because the *yama/niyama* form the moral and ethical foundation upon which all the other practices must rest, thus ensuring that any resulting accomplishments are used constructively for the good of the practitioner and everyone else.[40]

The Harmless Diet

Regarding the spiritual aspect of Gurudev's teachings on vegetarianism, the most pertinent of the *yama/niyama* is *ahimsa*, or nonviolence. In *The Healthy Vegetarian*, Gurudev declared: "Many people are concerned about the violence in our society and about the threat which that violence poses to the very existence of our planet. Our meat diet is a part of that violence. We should think about such things and about adopting a policy of *ahimsa*."[41]

As far as Gurudev was concerned, *ahimsa* doesn't simply mean nonkilling, because, in truth, it's impossible to live without destroying other lives. When we eat vegetables, we're killing; we're destroying living beings. What's more, even if we don't eat anything, we're still killing other organisms. When we drink water, we're killing millions of bacteria. When we breathe, we're killing millions of organisms. Gurudev told us that if it were only a matter of *killing*, he would advocate eating meat. After all, if we consider how many plants we must kill just to consume spinach during one meal, it would probably add up to 10 or 20 plants; but if we killed one sheep, say, or one cow, we could probably feed a number of people.

Consequently, if we think of killing as "sinful," we might feel that it's less sinful to kill one sheep or one cow than it is to kill many plants. So, it's not killing that we're referring to here. We're talking about *nonviolence*. As Gurudev expressed it, causing pain is violence. And if we want to be nonviolent with regard to our diet, then our food should come with as little pain as possible. We know, though, that plants are alive, too, and that they feel pain when we pick them and eat them. Why then should we eat plants and not eat meat?

In line with Gurudev's teachings, human beings, animals, plants, and even atoms have life, and in having life, we are all equal. Nonetheless, in the expression of consciousness, plants are not as developed as animals, and animals are not as developed as human beings. Human beings possess discrimination; we compare ourselves to other beings. Animals, on the other hand, don't compare themselves to us. Plants are even less developed when it comes to the expression of their consciousness. And the more developed the expression of consciousness in a particular life form, the more pain that organism feels when we destroy it. As Gurudev described it, "Cutting off the branch of a tree causes less pain than cutting off the limb of an animal."[42]

Undeniably, there have been a number of scientific studies demonstrating that plants do experience pain; but it is believed that they do not experience as much pain as animals do, because the consciousness of animals is more evolved. To confirm this conviction, Gurudev drew on the wisdom found in the Hindu scriptures, which say that consciousness sleeps in mineral life, dreams in plant life, and awakens in animal life. Thus, he taught that since we have to eat to live, and since we want to cause the least pain possible, we need to look to plants for sustenance. And, actually, we can inflict even less violence by eating only ripe fruits that fall from the tree. If we wait until the fruit or berry falls into our palm with the slightest touch of our hand, then we are not hurting the plant and are truly nonviolent. What's more, if we throw the seed somewhere on the ground when we finish the fruit, then we are helping to propagate the species, something that we can't do with animals.

Nature's Law

Gurudev believed that if people who ate meat visited a slaughterhouse and witnessed how the animals die, these individuals would never want to eat meat again. How many people, he wondered, would be able to bring an animal into their kitchen to kill it, to cut it open while it screamed and writhed in pain, to see its blood splashing everywhere, to clean up its fecal matter, and to cut up its flesh if there were no butchers available to do the job? His response to those who felt that it's humane to chop off the head of an animal quickly before it realizes that it's about to die was that this was certainly not the case. Why not? Because, he explained, by the process of thought transference, animals know that their death is imminent hours before the slaughter, even when they're miles away from the slaughterhouse.

Furthermore, it was ironic, he said, that there were so many animal rights organizations whose members advocated the protection of animals, yet those same people supported the killing of thousands of cows, calves, and other animals for their dinner parties, and so on. What's the difference, he questioned, between the life of their pet and the life of the cow, the lamb, or the pig that they eat? Even further, he warned that those who eat meat may think that they can get away with destroying the hearts and souls of millions of animals without facing the resulting *karma*, but in reality they cannot. Because even if they were not personally responsible for killing the animal, they contributed to the actions of those who did the killing and they share the *karma*. In keeping with Gurudev's Yogic approach, that which we do to other living beings eventually comes back to us. That, he stressed, is nature's law. And what's more, no one can save us from the workings of that law. In other words, *what we sow, we reap.* Gurudev's proposal: "Instead of eating animals, we should learn to love them or even to use them for good purposes, but not to kill and eat them. When you die, you have a graveyard somewhere. But, when they die, where is their graveyard? In your stomach."[43]

A gruesome image, no doubt. But one that can awaken us to the realization that when we eat the flesh of animals that have been slaughtered, we are absorbing the negative vibrations that emanate as a result of their terror and pain, effectively poisoning our system, because anything given carries the vibration of the giver. This is why, in the Hindu tradition, when a holy person offers you food, or any other item, the offering becomes purifying for the person who takes it, a sanctified object.

And then again, most people say that they want to live in a peaceful, loving world, but how can they cultivate a peaceful, loving environment if they themselves are filled with negative vibrations? As far as Gurudev was concerned, they cannot. That's why he used to say that our food should come to us as an offering of love, that whatever we eat should be the product of love. When he talked about food as a love offering, though, he wasn't referring to a chicken or fish or beef dish that someone lovingly offered.

What he meant was that we needed to ask ourselves: did the animal whose flesh became my food willingly and lovingly sacrifice itself for that purpose, for my sake? Of course, this question is rhetorical. Who can honestly imagine that an animal would willingly offer itself for destruction, to be slaughtered? Gurudev used to say, in fact, that the animals we kill actually hate us, adding that if the food we eat brings hatred into us, then we ourselves cannot develop love. Generally speaking, according to Yoga philosophy, it's not the food alone that can make us healthy and happy. To obtain the optimum benefit from our food—whether it be a gourmet meal or the most simple fare—that food needs to exude a positive vibration.

Even more remarkably, Gurudev indicated that if we become vegetarians, we can be certain that animals will actually worship us. He quoted the sage Thiruvalluvar, who said, "If a person refrains from killing to eat, such a one will be worshipped by all the creatures of the world." To illuminate this arcane notion, Gurudev explained that telecommunications is not only a human invention, but that animals also have their own method of telecommunication, which conveys good news as well as bad news. Therefore, if you save the life of any animal, other animals—even those of another species—will know. To shed even more light on this karmic phenomenon, he told us the following true story involving people whom he knew very well.

"Once, in India, a swami was invited to a rich man's house for a nice lunch. Normally, when the swami goes, a few disciples go with him. So they all went there and had a sumptuous lunch. It was served on beautiful silver plates, with silver cutlery, because the host was a very rich man. At the end of the meal, the swami blessed the man and his family, said good-bye, and left the house with his disciples.

"They had been walking for about half a mile when one disciple, the youngest one, came running to the swami: 'Swamiji, Swamiji, I made a terrible mistake!' The swami asked him, 'What mistake is that?'

" 'Oh, I'm even ashamed to tell you, because I have never done anything like this before!'

" 'It's alright,' the swami answered. 'Don't worry; tell me.' The disciple's hand was shaking as he pulled a silver spoon from his pocket. He said, 'I took this from the man's house!' The swami smiled at him and said, 'All right, you are still young; you are a beginner in spiritual practice. You will become strong as time goes on. Now, take it back and apologize; we will wait for you.'

"The other disciples questioned the swami: 'Why were you so lenient with him? Don't you think you should be stricter?' The swami said, 'No, it is not entirely his mistake.'

" 'He stole the spoon, and you say it's not his mistake?!'

"Finally, the swami explained, 'Do you know the fellow who fed us, the rich man? He collected all that money through theft. He was formerly a banker, and he used to overcharge his customers. So, in a way, he is a thief. When he fed us with his food, the vibrations of a thief also came with the food. You are all a little older and stronger, so it did not affect you. But he was affected by that vibration, so he took the spoon.' "[44]

The host in this anecdote was a thief, and the food that he served was bought with money that had been earned fraudulently. The food wasn't clean; it carried the negative vibration that came with thievery. This story teaches us that we need to be careful about how we get our food. Gurudev sought to make this point particularly clear with respect to eating animal food.

But Moses and Jesus Ate Meat!

Sometimes, people would argue with Gurudev that Moses and Jesus ate meat and fish. Whenever this argument came up, his rejoinder was: "Jesus walked on water; Jesus accepted crucifixion. Are you ready to do that? Moses spoke to God. Do you?" Usually, the debater would say, "Oh, I'm not like Jesus and Moses in that respect." And Gurudev would point out that when it comes to the great sages and saints, we think, "She did it; he did it; why can't I do it?" In truth, though, we merely choose certain aspects of their lives that we want to follow. To illustrate this fact, Gurudev used to recount a story about the renowned Hindu saint Acharya Shankara.

Once, on a hot day, the holy man was walking with his students. He was very thirsty, so when he saw a man walking in their direction who was holding a pot of some kind of liquid, he stopped the man and asked if he could have a drink. The man, hesitating, said that he didn't think that what he had was fit for a holy man (it was a type of regional liquor). Shankara told him that it didn't matter and that he would take some. His students were thirsty too, so they also drank from the pot. When the group continued to walk, the disciples were not able walk in a straight line; drunk from the liquor, they were weaving here and there, all over the road.

After walking a few more miles in the hot sun, Shankara was thirsty again. This time, he noticed a shop at the side of the road where a black-smith was boiling lead in a pot. The liquid was milky and white, so Shankara said, "Hmm, you seem to be boiling some milk." And without even giving the blacksmith a chance to say a word, he picked up the pot and drank some of the liquid. Then, he looked over at his disciples and said, "I think that you all must be thirsty, too. Come on, drink!" His students immediately recognized their mistake, and they fell at his feet. They realized that they couldn't imitate everything that their master did.

Gurudev often quoted from the biblical scriptures when discussing veg-etarianism as the natural diet for human beings. He referred, for example, to Genesis 1:29 in the Bible, where God says, "Behold, I have given you every herb-bearing seed which is upon the face of the earth, and every tree in which are fruits; for you it shall be as meat." He also quoted the Dead Sea Scrolls, which contain some of the teachings on meat eating from the time of Jesus: "And the flesh of slain beasts in a person's body will become his own tomb. For I tell you truly, he who kills, kills himself, and whosoever eats the flesh of slain beasts eats the body of death." And he alluded to St. Paul, too, who said in his letters to the Romans, "It is good not to eat flesh . . ." (Romans 14:2).

Additionally, Gurudev had the opportunity to read some of the works of fourteenth-century Christian saints from manuscripts housed in the library of the Order of the Cross, in England. He said that almost every one of them recommended eating pure vegetarian food and abstaining from liquor. He recalled that some of the saints even laughed at those who ate meat and drank wine in the name of the Eucharist, asking them how they expected their minds to be clean if they ate meat and drank alcohol.[45] And, he explained, it is essentially for this reason, to make our minds pure, that almost every religion advocates at least some days of adherence to a vegetarian diet. He noted that, whether they know the reasons or not, religious people of many faiths stay away from animal food on auspicious days. Why? Because by staying away from meat, you make a day holy. From Gurudev's point of view, if you stay away from meat every day, then every day will be a holy day.

Our Choice: Compassion or Cupidity

In *The Healthy Vegetarian*, which was published in 1986, Gurudev wrote, "Our human family is starving in many parts of the world." To those who argued that overpopulation is the cause of starvation in some parts of the world, he countered: "I say that overpopulation is not the problem; rather, human greed is the problem. If we were only willing to care and share, there would be enough for everyone."[46]

Today, 24 years later, the situation hasn't changed. Indeed, in this era of worldwide greed and corruption, as well as unspeakable violence perpetrated against some of our planet's most vulnerable citizens, it seems certain that hunger and starvation are even more widespread. What's more, the voracious appetite for meat, a commodity that many societies view as a status symbol, guarantees that countless human beings, including millions of children, will suffer from malnutrition and die from starvation. Gurudev clearly understood that a meat-based diet contributed directly to the tragedy of world hunger. Addressing this issue in his talks, he stated that in order to get 1 pound of meat, farmers need to feed 16 pounds of grain to 1 steer. Moreover, the amount of grain that farmers use to produce meat almost equals the amount consumed as food in poorer countries.

To make matters even clearer, in *The Healthy Vegetarian*, Gurudev included the following statistics cited in Frances Moore Lappé's book, *Diet for a Small Planet*: 1 acre of land used to produce grain provides 5 times more protein than an acre used to produce meat; 1 acre of beans or lentils provides 10 times more protein; and an acre of vegetables, 15 times more protein.[47]

Obviously, it takes a great deal more land to feed a meat-eater than it does to feed a vegetarian. From the standpoint of Gurudev's teachings, land belongs to everyone. This doesn't mean that we shouldn't possess land to use for personal gain, but it does mean that we do have the choice to use the land to feed only ourselves or our fellow citizens or to utilize the land for the good of the larger human community. In his commentary on *sutra* 37 in Book II of the *Yoga Sutras*—"To one established in nonstealing, all wealth comes"—Gurudev wrote: "What is grown in the United States can first be given to its citizens, with the surplus divided among everyone else. If we know how to care and share, no poverty or hunger need exist anywhere."[48] And as he pointed out in *The Healthy*

Vegetarian, if everyone were to become a vegetarian, there would be plenty of food—and plenty of protein—for all. In the same text, he cited Mahatma Gandhi, who said: "The earth has enough for everyone's need but not enough for everyone's greed."[49] No doubt Gurudev would have agreed with the *Mahaparinirvana Sutra*, an ancient Buddhist text, which declares that eating meat destroys the attitude of great compassion.

On the other hand, we can't expect everyone to be a vegetarian. As I mentioned earlier, sometimes it's impossible for people to follow a vegetarian diet. Would we expect, for example, everyone living in Alaska or in Tibet to give up eating meat? How would they survive if there were nothing else available? Gurudev's response to such questions was unambiguous: If, for some reason, you have no choice but to eat meat to survive, then, without a doubt, you must do it. "In such a situation," he counseled, "you can at least feel grateful to the animal whose life was sacrificed."[50]

CONCLUSION: AN ATTITUDE OF GRATITUDE

In the beginning of this article, I pointed out that Gurudev viewed the benefits of vegetarianism holistically, from the physical, mental, and spiritual perspectives. He taught that our body is a vegetarian body; that we are naturally vegetarians; and that vegetarianism is the key to optimum health. He described how the mind is affected by what we put into the body, how particular foods make the mind restless or dull or balanced. And he made it clear that vegetarianism promotes and supports spiritual growth by helping us develop and express compassion for and gratitude toward all sentient beings. As he saw it, "The aim of Yoga is to go back to nature as much as possible. To lead a natural life, with simple food, simple dress, simple living."[51] He used to tell us that when we lead a natural life, our mind will become elevated, and it will be easy to solve global problems. We will be grateful for all that we have. And we will be willing to share with those who are in need.

To help his disciples cultivate and sustain an attitude of gratitude, Gurudev recommended that they recite the following prayer before meals:

OM Beloved Mother Nature,
You are here on our table as our food;
You are endlessly bountiful, benefactress of all;
Please grant us health and strength,
Wisdom and dispassion
To find permanent peace and joy;
Mother Nature is my mother;
My father is the Lord of All;

All the people are my relatives;
The entire universe is my home.
I offer this unto OM, that Truth which is universal.
May the entire universe be filled with Peace and Joy, Love and Light.
May the Light of Truth overcome all darkness.
Victory to that Light!

I end this essay with gratitude, grateful to have had the opportunity to share Gurudev's teachings on vegetarianism and to convey some aspects of his broad and deep knowledge of the ancient science of Yoga. Quoting Lord Krishna in the *Bhagavad Gita*, he wrote in *The Healthy Vegetarian*: "Yoga is not for the person who eats too much, nor for the one who fasts excessively." And in his own words: "Going to extremes can sometimes be easier, but the middle path is what we need for a life of health and peace. Let us think in a peaceful way; eat in a peaceful way. Let all of our actions be done in this spirit."[52]

Sri Gurudev Swami Satchidananda attained *mahasamadhi* (the passing of an enlightened being) in South India on August 18, 2002. Having accepted invitations to participate in a peace conference and to attend a film premiere, he flew to Chennai, the capital of Tamil Nadu. Nearly 88 years old, he was still actively serving at home and abroad, traveling at a pace that would challenge those who were decades younger. He had the energy to maintain such a schedule because he had complete faith that he was an instrument of the Divine, because he was filled with unconditional love for all beings, because he was committed to selfless service, and because his mind was always peaceful and his body pure and strong. In short, he practiced what he preached. And like all genuine spiritual teachers, his attitude was: This is what I know from my experience. If you like my advice, follow it. If you don't, let it go.

NOTES

1. Sita Bordow et al., *Sri Swami Satchidananda: Apostle of Peace* (Buckingham: Integral Yoga Publications, 1986), 3–45.
2. The Phrase Finder. http://www.phrases.org/uk/meanings/index.html (accessed December 1, 2009).
3. University of Adelaide. University of Adelaide Library. http://eBooks@ Adelaide.edu.au (accessed December 1, 2009).
4. The Phrase Finder. http://www.phrases.org/uk/meanings/index.html (accessed December 1, 2009).
5. Ibid.
6. Sita Bordow, *Apostle of Peace*, 203–216.
7. Ibid., 217–219.

8. Ibid., 220–240.

9. Ibid., 244.

10. Sri Swami Satchidananda, *The Healthy Vegetarian* (Buckingham: Integral Yoga Publications, 1986), v–vii.

11. Sri Swami Satchidananda, Talk, August 11, 1987 (Buckingham, VA: Satchidananda Ashram-Yogaville Archives).

12. Ibid., *The Healthy Vegetarian*, vii.

13. Ibid., vii–viii.

14. Ibid., 5.

15. Ibid., 5–6.

16. Ibid., 7–9.

17. Ibid., 8.

18. Ibid.

19. Sri Swami Satchidananda, Talk, June 9, 1990 (Buckingham, VA: Satchidananda Ashram-Yogaville Archives).

20. Sri Swami Satchidananda, *The Healthy Vegetarian*, 23–24.

21. Ibid., 36–37.

22. Sri Swami Satchidnanda, Talk, May 13, 1989 (Buckingham, VA: Satchidananda AshramYogaville Archives).

23. Sri Swami Satchidananda, Talk, November 14, 1988 (Buckingham, VA: Satchidananda Ashram-Yogaville Archives).

24. Sri Swami Satchidananda, Talk, August 12, 1989 (Buckingham, VA: Satchidananda Ashram-Yogaville Archives).

25. Sri Swami Satchidananda, Talk, June 22, 2002 (Buckingham, VA: Satchidananda Ashram-Yogaville Archives).

26. Sri Swami Satchidananda, *The Healthy Vegetarian*, 35.

27. Ibid., 36.

28. Ibid., 28.

29. Ibid., 28.

30. Ibid., 31–32.

31. Ibid., 33.

32. Ibid., 38–42.

33. Ibid., 38–41.

34. Sri Patanjali, *Yoga Sutras of Patanjali*, trans. and commentary by Sri Swami Satchidananda, 10th ed. Buckingham, VA: Integral Yoga Publications, 2004, 28.

35. Sri Swami Satchidananda, *The Living Gita* (Buckingham: Integral Yoga Publications, 1988), 249.

36. Ibid., 250.

37. Ibid., 251.

38. Ibid., 252.

39. Sri Patanjali, *Yoga Sutras*, xiii.

40. Ibid., 125.

41. Sri Swami Satchidananda, *The Healthy Vegetarian*, 10.

42. Ibid., 11.

43. Ibid., 14.

44. Ibid., 15.

45. Ibid., 17–18.

46. Ibid., 16.

47. Ibid., 16.

48. Sri Patanjali, *Yoga Sutras*, 134–35.

49. Sri Swami Satchidananda, *The Healthy Vegetarian*, 16.

50. Rev. Sandra Kumari de Sachy, *Bound to be Free: The Liberating Power of Prison Yoga* (Buckingham: Integral Yoga Publications, 2010), 219.

51. Sri Swami Satchidananda, *The Healthy Vegetarian*, 54.

52. Ibid., 55.

6

From Darkness to Light: Vegetarianism and the Yogi's Emergence into Clear Perception

Natalie J. Ullmann

Patanjali's *Yoga Sutra* 1.1: *atha yoganushashanam*

"Now (at this point of transition) the exposition of yoga."[1]

Patanjali's *Yoga Sutra* 1.2: *yogash chitta-vritti-nirodha*

"Yoga is the suppression of the fluctuations of the mind."[2]

"The problem is that you won't really be able to understand why eating meat is an obstacle in your practice until you stop eating it." The statement was offered gently, or so I thought. The student had been defending the lifestyle of the carnivorous Yogi as I walked up to the group, and the other teachers had redirected her comments in my direction.

"But I'm on the path, I'm making progress," her defensive tone and unwillingness to make eye contact not seeming concordant with making progress in Yoga. *Sutra* 2.46 of Patanjali's *Yoga Sutra*, an authoritative ancient text on Yoga, suggests that ease, or *sukham*, is a significant dimension of *asana* practice. Some result must have been apparent, or she would not have continued practicing, and yet, she did not seem at ease.

"The practice of *ahimsa*, or nonviolence, is given very prominent placement in the teachings, so we have to assume that placement is not arbitrary," I responded. "As long as we continue to ingest food from an animal who has suffered, on some level our perceptual mechanisms must remain shut down and unaware or we would feel the animal's suffering; we would know it as our own. This closing off of our awareness impedes our progress on the path. When we are aware, to continue to ingest such suffering would be unthinkable." A look of shock and sadness arose in her eyes, which quickly hardened as she turned brusquely and walked away.

In the second century CE a Yoga adept by the name of Patanjali produced an authoritative treatise on the practices of Yoga commonly referred to as Patanjali's *Yoga Sutra*. The text provides a framework of the methods of Yoga, as well as a terminology with which to discuss the goals of the practice. Patanjali declares the state of Yoga to be the experience where one's essential, or pure spiritual, nature prevails over the tendencies of the mind (*vrittis*). Until that moment occurs, one will experience self and world as a reflection of those tendencies. Patanjali's *Yoga Sutra* delineates a systematic method of dismantling the power of the *vrittis*, allowing Yogins to identify with their essential nature.

> Patanjali's *Yoga Sutra* 4.3: *nimittam-aprayojakam prakritinam varana-bhedas tu tatah kshetrikavat*
>
> "Good and bad deeds are not the direct causes in the transformations of nature, but they act as breakers of obstacles to the evolutions—as a farmer breaks the obstacles to the course of water, which then runs down by its own nature."—Swami Vivekananda[3]

YOGA AND THE DEVELOPMENT OF CLEAR PERCEPTION

> Patanjali's *Yoga Sutra* 2.28: *yoganganusthanad asuddhi kshaye jnana diptir avivika khyateh*
>
> "Through practicing the [eight] limbs of yoga—upon the diminishing of impurities—there is a light of knowing, [leading] up to *viveka-khyata*, the identification of *viveka* [discriminitive wisdom]"[4]

The methods of Yoga are empirical, systematic, and designed to be replicated. The efficacy of the methodology has been confirmed through experience by countless Yogins for thousands of years. As in a chemistry experiment where a minute detail left out or shifted in sequence can alter the results completely, the methodology of Yoga has been cultivated to obtain self-realization—and a minute detail, left out of one's Yoga practice, will alter the results that one obtains. Contemporary practitioners are quick to adopt the methods of Yoga for the enjoyment of personal lifestyle appetites: consumerism, social cravings, short-term stress reduction, and other transient and insubstantial gains. In exchanging the formal structure of the method for a fractional snippet of immediate gratification, the promise of stable well-being and deep satisfaction intrinsic to the deeper processes of Yoga is forfeited.

While much of Patanjali's text concerns the subtle focus and surrender cultivated in meditation, in the second chapter of the *Yoga Sutra*, Patanjali specifies the external actions required to support the internal dynamics of the practice. These powerful practices are called the "*yamas.*" The *yamas* are the "*mahavratam,*" or great vows of the Yogi. There is no condition under which they are not applicable.[5] Before *asana*, before meditation, before *pranayama*, before even cultivating a fervent desire for success in the practice,[6] the Yogin is advised to renounce all harmful behavior. In other words, the journey to the true clarity and peace which is yoga *begins* with the renunciation of all animal food. *Ahimsa*, or nonharming, cannot properly be practiced without this dietary restriction, as there is no animal food obtained, whether it be flesh food or honey, that does not cause pain, either through literal taking of the life, or through enslavement.[7] Eating is, for many, the most frequently harmful behavior in which they engage. The ongoing partaking of food obtained at the expense of the life of another is a continual erroneous reinforcement of the fear-based misperception that one must harm others in order to survive. To practice Yoga while consuming animal products is much like digging a hole only to fill it up again, over and over.

THE PRIMARY FORMS OF VRITTIS

Patanjali's Yoga Sutra 1.5: *vrittaha panchatayyah klishtaklishtah*

"There are five primary forms of *vrittis*, and they either obstruct our clarity, causing pain (*klishtah*) or they do not (*aklishtah*)."[8]

Patanjali's *Yoga Sutra* 1.6: *pramana-viparyaya-vikalpa-nidra-smritayah*

"They are right knowledge, wrong knowledge, verbal delusion, sleep and memory."

Indoctrination in food paradigms begins at an early age, when the freedom to make individual choices is minimal at best. This indoctrination is the basis for many of the *vrittis*. The depth of the influence of conditioning about food and the influence of what we eat on our state of mind is evidenced by the difficulty many aspiring practitioners encounter when the desire to shift to a violence-free diet arouses deep states of conflict within the context of family, spiritual groups, friends, and love relationships. To change what we eat is directly connected to a deep shift in identity and values. If I am no longer eating what my friends eat, what tribe will I belong to? To choose to eat in such a way that breaks out of our culture and places the well-being of all beings on par with our social group makes a profound statement. All living beings are as valuable as those with whom we are the most intimate. To take on such a primal shift is to break down our most fundamental tendencies. When this behavior is adopted in its classical placement at the initial stages of practice, it is a powerful catalyst for transformation that allows the following stages of work to proceed more quickly.

Patanjali identifies five primary *vrittis*—right knowledge, wrong knowledge, verbal delusion, sleep, and memory. When these *vrittis* are not suppressed through proper practice their dominance in the mind-field colors our experience of the world.

RIGHT KNOWLEDGE

Patanjali's *Yoga Sutra* 1.7: *pratyakshanumanagamah pramanani*

"Valid means of knowledge are direct perception, inference, and testimony."[9]

Let me begin with a story: Splash! Down into the water we went. The dive master plunged deeper and encouraged us remain close by on this, our first, underwater adventure. Sunlight scattered through a sea that appeared to be a brilliant blue green, but the water was clear, absolutely clear. With the exception of the outcropping of the reef ahead, the ocean floor was a barren wasteland. Inflated by the conquest of this alien environment, our little scuba group darted to and fro celebrating the liberating experience of this new frontier. And then, unencumbered by tanks (or for that matter arms and legs), and adorned with shimmering scales of many colors, the sovereign inhabitants of the sea kingdom revealed themselves. Silent and lovely, the tiny school of fish glided towards us with an innate dignity and grace that no earthly title could confer. By comparison, I felt foolish and clumsy, masquerading as a sea creature with rubber fins, tank, and wet suit. Pride crumbled into humility, remembering that such beautiful beings were held prisoners in tanks, in the homes and offices of others of my kind. Surprise, wonder and delight arose with the experience of their obvious sentience when interacted with in their proper abode. How humbling it was, to realize that my perception of these grand creatures had been so tainted by their behavior when in captivity. As if any being could ever express its true nature when confined in a cage or a tank.

Emerging onto the land of concrete, we shed our rubber skins. A dinner celebration had been planned to honor this, our first brave dive into the sea. Appetites fully engaged, we went in ardent pursuit of the finest eatery above sea level. Our chosen venue was opulent, magnificently lit and very expensive. The special of the day was a tantalizing mix of the ocean's most delectable beings, prepared especially to delight the human palate. The waitress, glowing with pride at her offering, placed the platter in front of me. My anticipation of a delicious meal dissolved in a flood of tears, and then more tears. In a moment of clarity the connection between the meal placed before me, and the beautiful beings I had played with a short time before, had been revealed.

How strange that my friends and I could be so confused that we could swim and play with the fishes and then, to celebrate, plan a party where we would eat them. An acquaintance once told me she had a similar experience on a dive trip—and since then has never eaten fish after a scuba dive. One wonders, if she cannot eat fish after a scuba dive, how she ever eats it at all.

* * *

What is right knowledge? Well, according to Patanjali right knowledge has three dimensions; it is based on correct perception, correct deduction, and scriptural authority. For the non-Yogis, their most immediate source of information would most likely be what they experience, what they figure out based on what they experience, and recognized authority, which is most often science. All of these things fluctuate. Just as in the story above, what we see or feel or know to be true can change from moment to moment.

Even testimony based on scientific research, which is often used to validate a carnivorous lifestyle, is continually changing. The term "paradigm" was coined by Thomas Kuhn to signify a structure of agreements upon which the dominant scientific model of any given period is based. In other words, we're talking about the underlying beliefs that shape the scientific development at any given point in time, or we could say "scientific *vrittis*." According to Kuhn, the research that is advocated will support the dominant paradigm of the time, and that which does not fall into alignment with the dominant paradigm is disregarded. A scientific revolution is characterized by the overturning of one or more of these underlying models. For many years, scientists and philosophers built their work on the paradigm that the Sun revolved around the Earth. Copernicus' radical assertion that in fact the Earth moved was met with denial and controversy. Just as philosophers and scientists of Copernicus's day were operating under the heavy hand of the Catholic Church, much of modern scientific research into food is financed by those with a vested interest in keeping the general population carnivorous.[10]

Back to our story: Sylvia Earle, former chief scientist of the U.S. National Oceanic and Atmospheric Administration, has written, "[Fish] are our fellow citizens with scales and fins. . . . I would never eat anyone I know personally, I wouldn't eat a grouper any more than I'd eat a cocker spaniel. They're so good-natured, so curious. You know, fish are sensitive, they have personalities, they hurt when they are wounded."[11]

WRONG KNOWLEDGE

Patanjali's *Yoga Sutra* 1.8: *viparyayo mithya-jnanam a tad rupa pratishtham*

"Mistaken knowledge is an idea which is not based on the nature or form of its object."

The air was full of the sounds of chairs scraping and cars whizzing by. We were in a small town, but it might have been Manhattan, the sounds were so penetrating. After 10 days of silent meditation, the ear becomes very sensitized. This waitress was not beaming cordially; she was gruff and rushed. It was brunch time at the most popular diner in the village. We were laughing and sharing, absorbing the wonder of reemerging into a cacophonous world after resting in deep silence—everything around us was vibrating. Our appetites had been reduced to the barest essentials by the simple vegetarian fare on the retreat—and now, freedom of choice! We eagerly opened the menus. It was a step back into the life we led before the retreat—full of television, phone calls, chatter, and savory edibles. After a moment, one of my companions furrowed his brow and exclaimed, "Wait, that vow we took, not to kill, that doesn't include what we eat, does it?" He looked seriously concerned—this question was not frivolous. The enthusiasm at the reintroduction of decadence into our lives was immediately stifled. Every choice on the menu, had, at one time or another, obviously had a mother.

"No. It means that you shouldn't kill anything yourself—like you shouldn't kill a spider," piped up another member of the group.

"Do you really think it matters whether you kill the animal yourself or not? It's still dead," I responded.

Another group member chimed in, "Well, I have a friend whose brother has a guru, and the guru told him that he should eat meat."

I pondered momentarily how to point out that this mysterious guru, who we did not know, was addressing the needs of a specific individual whose circumstances we did not know.

"I don't know who that guru was, or why they said that, but I do know this: we can say we are choosing NOT to observe 'Thou shalt not kill' and then eat meat, but we cannot say that eating meat is not killing."

The thoughtful silence was broken by the waitress' welcome arrival to take our orders. The fellow who asked the question chuckled warmly, raised his eyebrows and pronounced, "We'll have five orders of toast please!"

* * *

The paradigm of wrong knowledge is supported when we do not investigate what lies underneath the level of our immediate experience. Another way to understand this *sutra* is that what we experience is disconnected from what's actually happening. It is interesting that we can acknowledge that we shouldn't kill something but then perceive that our action in eating flesh food does not involve taking the life of another. Clearly, if we are purchasing and consuming flesh food, we are creating the market for murder, in the same way that any other consumer behavior establishes a market for that which is being purchased.

This disconnection is further reflected in the public's general denial of the relationship between the consumption of flesh food and early death. The statistics supporting the connection between the consumption of meat and dairy products and mortality rate is so extensive it is beyond the scope of this chapter, but still the illusion that a meat-based diet is healthy persists in the public eye.

Note this small summary from Howard Lyman's *Mad Cowboy*:

> The German Cancer Research Center conducted a study of over 1,900 vegetarians, and found that rates for all forms of cancer were only 56% of the normal rate. The aforementioned study of Seventh Day Adventist men also found that this group, about half of whom are vegetarian, and who eat, on average about 50% more fiber than the general population, suffers 55% less prostrate cancer than other American males. Similarly, a ten-year-study of over 120,000 Japanese men reported that vegetarian men had a lower incidence of prostrate cancer than meat eaters.[12]

It is interesting to note that not only do we dwell in incorrect knowledge that deludes us into believing that we do not kill when we eat meat; we dwell in incorrect knowledge about the manner in which this choice impacts us.

VERBAL DELUSION

Patanjali's *Yoga Sutra* 1.9: *shabda-jnanupati vastu-sunyo vikalpah.*

"Fancy is the notion called into being by mere words, having nothing to answer to it in reality."[13]

The lesson had gone over, I thought, particularly well. It was the first time that I had introduced the concept of veganism and Yoga with a group in a suburban setting, and they had stayed open and listened for the whole teaching. The community was clearly, by and large, well-educated and intelligent. By their response, it was apparent it was something they had given some thought to previously, and after the class I was approached by many with sincere and heartfelt questions.

"But of course, Natalie, there is Compassionate Killing, this is one alternative," the student was a wise and compassionate woman, with a long history of successful public service. Her comment startled me.

"Compassionate killing?" I said. "There is no such thing; it's an oxymoron. I'll tell you what, we'll put you up in a fancy mansion, feed you tempting healthy morsels to fatten you up and then when it suits us, we'll kill you. Is that compassion?" Her face changed abruptly as she realized what she had said, and what I had said. "Oh, I see what you mean," she nodded.

* * *

A label is a powerful thing. When someone tells us that a person is stupid or smart or funny or corrupt, the power of that statement, made in the absence of personal experience, creates a tendency for us to perceive that person in a particular way. It takes work on our part to get beyond these labels. We may never get to know the person well enough that we discover who they are on a deeper level. Immersed in advertising, labels bombard us on all sides; removing ourselves from their influence is very difficult. We are so used to misrepresentation that, on one level we stop interpreting the information: new and improved, homemade, natural flavors are all terms that advertisers have concocted and used until the terms have become devoid of meaning. The term Compassionate Agriculture is a marketing tool, designed to create the impression that something is more palatable, safer, or less harmful than it truly is. But this is not new; seldom do you hear animal foods called exactly what they are, the decaying flesh of a once living, breathing, feeling being. The truth is obscured by polite euphemisms. We are given images that do not correspond at all to the reality of what is happening—we buy into the idea of happy cows on farms. Or we call ourselves vegetarians when in fact we are still eating fish. We call ourselves vegans when we still nip an egg or two, politely deluding ourselves that we are not harming others, all the while ignoring the fact that fish are not vegetables, neither are eggs; and compassionate killing could never occur in the context of mass production and a consumer market.

SLEEP

Patanjali's *Yoga Sutra* 1.10: *abhava-pratyayalambana vritiire nidra*

"Sleep (*nidra*) is a thought pattern that has as its object inertia or blankness."[14]

"Wake up!" my friend shouted, laughing as I stepped out into the street oblivious to oncoming traffic and the big orange hand on the crosswalk sign. Chagrined, I stepped back on the sidewalk, I mean, what kind of a Yoga teacher was I anyway, to be so unconscious. We were headed out to eat in a very carnivorous community. Our choices were limited to one restaurant, which offered one option for the non-meat eater. Entering the venue, I must admit to feeling a little queasy at the smell. But then, it was a restaurant in an unfamiliar culture—so yes, the smells were strange. Ignoring it, we ordered chips and guacamole, and my friend ordered a bowl of soup. The topic turned to vegetarianism and its relationship Yoga. Our orders arrived and we relaxed into conversation.

"Yoga requires that one come into total awareness, beyond the field of normal perception. And the thing is, whenever we consume animal food, we have to shut off a bit of our awareness. Part of our awareness has to become unconscious; we have to go to sleep. If we were completely aware we would feel what that animal was feeling as they were milked or forcibly impregnated or slaughtered. We would experience it directly. How could one continue to eat these things in such a state? It would be very difficult."

I paused in my soliloquy long enough to consider my friend. As I looked in her direction, I noticed that she was staring at her soup with a look of revulsion. Oh, no. I had spoiled her meal.

"I'm sorry, did this conversation upset you?"

"No," she said, "I am worried about what's in this soup." I didn't know how to respond, initiating a conversation about food and awareness during a meal was perhaps a thoughtless choice. "Well, have some guacamole." She responded: "I'm worried about what is in the guacamole, too." She really looked sad.

The waitress came and took the soup away. My friend turned to me and said, "I think there was pig skin in that soup." Pig skin? I was suddenly worried about what was in the guacamole too. How did she even recognize it as pig skin? I didn't want to know. As we sent the waitress away with the unfinished guacamole, I reflected on how easy it had been to turn off that perception of the funny smell when we walked in. Of course it was a funny smell. It was animal food. And we had deliberately turned away from the perception.

* * *

The fourth of the modifications that Patanjali address is *nidra*, commonly translated as the Yogic state of deep meditation, which resembles sleep (the literal meaning of the word). In Yoga, this is the instance where the mind turns away from the external world. But the word *nidra* may also be translated as slothful from drowsiness or darkness.[15] And clearly we have moments when we dwell not in right knowledge or wrong knowledge, but just in a fog that obscures what is happening around us. When we are drowsy, we are not paying attention. In the dark, we cannot see. Some conditions are conducive to physical sleep. When the lights are low, the music quiet, and the room warm we are inclined to go into drowsy unconsciousness. Likewise, when we are fixed in a view of the world, encountering something that we don't want to experience may result in a shut down of our perceptual mechanisms. An extreme example could be fainting from shock.

Such is the paradox of the factory farm: they are often invisible, the animals confined out of sight, the waste from the animals sloughed off away from the farm and into our waterways.[16] As we drive through the bucolic landscapes of rural America, it is easy to turn our awareness away from what is politely not mentioned. "What agribusiness? It's beautiful here." When the suffering of animals is hidden behind the pristine outer walls of an animal confinement center, we do not need to consider the squeals of distress that go on within those walls. To consider that would be to wake up to the experience that the commodities in question were really sentient beings with thoughts and feelings. Pigs, for example, have been known to have one of the highest IQs of all animals.[17] One has to wonder what it must be like for such an intelligent animal to live its life confined without sunlight or room to move or take any kind of voluntary action at all. Consider this, if we were to take the most intelligent humans on the planet, and confine them in tiny rooms with no windows, without sensory stimulation at all, for the entirety of their lives. What would their life-experience be like?

To ignore, to turn away, to cultivate ignorance, creates more ignorance. We are adept at ignoring the consequences of our animal food consumption on our bodies, the planet and our souls. Even when it arises momentarily in our sensory consciousness, we tune out the questions that arise and go quickly back to sleep.

MEMORY

Patanjali's Yoga Sutra 1.11: *anabhuta-vishayasampramoshah smritih*

"Memory is not allowing those matters of enjoyment or experience to be forgotten."[18]

"I love Thanksgiving!" the student in the front row exclaimed gleefully.

I had been speaking about the annual Jivamukti Thanksgiving retreat. Members of the tribe gather annually at Ananda Ashram in Monroe, New York, to celebrate and give thanks for the present moment, the lives we have, and the earth itself and the love to be shared among all creatures. This celebration of peaceful thanks begins each year with a delicious savory vegan meal: sage-scented tofu, vegan mashed potatoes, sauteed greens, and the like. I had been advocating the escape from the usual Thanksgiving celebration to join us for this celebration, free of violence.

The student thoughtfully pursed her lips, shook her head, and said, "We always have a nonviolent Thanksgiving. Our family never fights, we love one another very much and enjoy getting to see one another."

"Does your family serve turkey for Thanksgiving?"

"Yes, of course; it's a tradition!"

I considered a moment before responding, "Well, then, you are not having a nonviolent Thanksgiving, right?" She was clearly jarred by my statement. I had disturbed this peaceful recollection of a happy event in her life. But then, that recollection of the happiness experienced obscured the clear perception of the celebration.

* * *

An estimated 46 million turkeys were slaughtered for Thanksgiving in 2009.[19] That's approximately one-sixth of the population of the entire United States.[20] One can imagine the outrage if such a slaughter of human beings were to take place in such a short period of time. We are attached to our happy memories of this holiday from our childhoods, but those memories lack clarity. When we step back a bit and consider the turkey slaughter we can see that a party around a stuffed turkey is a party around a corpse. The continued celebration in this manner reinforces the memory and obscures our ability to perceive clearly.

We could just as well have a party, a new kind of party, without the turkey.

The fifth of the *vrittis* identified by Patanjali is memory, or *smrtih*. In its most obvious sense, it refers to the waves of memory that we notice during meditation. We sit quietly and then an image or sensation arises from our past and drifts through our consciousness. When we consider the *vrittis* as a tendency, a memory becomes an ingrained idea of who we are. This obliterates the experience of Yoga and confines us. One of the greatest conflicts I see in students is that they are often kind people, compassionate people who are completely unaware that their food choices are unkind. Their whole lives they have learned the societal norms for "niceness," all the while dining on the flesh of their animal brethren and consuming products obtained through the enslavement of other sentient beings. It's confusing, to say the least, to reach adulthood and have it revealed to you that eating meat is brutal and violent, and that it is not necessary. No one, at least by the time they get to a Yoga class, is deliberately seeking to behave unkindly.

The images of happy cows are seared in our memories, obscuring the reality of mass production that demands forced impregnation and the treatment of sentient beings as though they were commodities to be manufactured. To dive underneath these illusory memories of apparent goodness, which conceal the current, disturbing state of affairs, demands a reevaluation our past actions in light of this new information. Maybe we aren't as nice as we think we are. To go this deeply and honestly into self-examination is an excruciating piece of internal work. But, to be free, to be in Yoga, is to be fully in the present moment, liberated from the ingrained perceptions accumulated from past experience and able to make conscious aware choices in every circumstances. As a veteran of the pharmaceutical industry, I struggled deeply with my own inner conflict about my past, until my teacher turned to me one day before class and said, "Well, Natalie, whatever it is we did, it couldn't have been too bad, because we are here now."

The student we started the article discussing was doing her practice, but the depth of her transformation was not apparent. Or at least not as apparent as the transformations I had witnessed in those who had embraced a plant-based diet and the practice of *ahimsa* wholeheartedly. The renunciation of animal food is truly a small sacrifice to make in exchange for the expanse of possibility that arises as the Yogi moves towards the state of freedom that is Yoga: a state beyond constructs, unbound by the fear, worry, depression, and sense of inadequacy we've been conditioned to accept. Perhaps we are free, but there is always an opportunity to be freer. Perhaps we have been loving to others, but there is always an opportunity to be more loving. Perhaps we have been kind. But there is always an opportunity to be kinder. Yoga is not about judging the past. Rather, it is an opportunity to move more deeply into each moment as it arises, as we move into the future.

NOTES

1. Zambita, Salvatore, *The Unadorned Thread of Yoga, The Yoga-Sutra of Patanjali in English, A Compilation of English Translations of Sri Patanjali's Exposition of the Yoga Darshana*, Poulsbo (Washington: The Yoga Sutras Institute Press, 1992), p. 10.

2. Ibid., p. 12.

3. Ibid., p. 351.

4. Houston, Vyaas, *The Yoga Sutra Workbook: The Certainty of Freedom* (Warwick, New York: American Sanskrit Institute, 1995), 11.28.

5. Zambita, *Unadorned Thread of Yoga*, p. 176. Patanjali's *Yoga Sutra* 2.31 *eta jati-desa-kala-samayanavacchinnah sarva-bhauma mahavratam*. These great vows are applicable to all levels and spheres irrespective of circumstance, time, place and birth.

6. In the limb that follows the restraints, the *niyamas*, one is advised to cultivate passion or intensity in their practice. This step is indicated AFTER the

yamas. We might consider that the practice of the *yamas*, and *ahimsa* renders that passion or intensity conducive to spiritual growth, rather than distracting.

7. The point is often raised that even plants feel pain, and that small animals and insects may be killed in the process of harvesting plant crops. However, the raising of animals for food creates suffering of both the animals and the plants (and sometimes other animals) that they eat. When we restrict our diet to plant food we do the least amount of harm to the least amount of beings.

8. Zambita, *Unadorned Thread of Yoga,* p. 18.

9. Ibid., p. 22.

10. The Harvard School of Public Health. http://www.hsph.harvard.edu/nutritionsource/what-should-you-eat/pyramid/.

11. Will Tuttle, Ph.D., *The World Peace Diet,* Lantern Books, 2005, p. 107.

12. Lyman, Howard and Merzer, Glenn, "Mad Cowboy, The Plain Truth from the Cattle Farmer who won't eat Meat," Scribner, 1998, p. 31. Chapter Two of this book is an excellent review of the literature on the correlations between the consumption of animal products and mortality rates.

13. Zambita, *Unadorned Thread of Yoga,* p. 27, translation by Dvivedi.

14. Ibid., p. 29, translation adapted from Jnaneshvara.

15. Cologne Digital Sanskrit Lexicon http://webapps.uni-koeln.de/cgi-bin/tamil/recherche.

16. Scully, Matthew, Dominion, *The Power of Man, the Suffering of Animals,* St. Martin's Press, 2002, p. 258.

17. Robbins, John, *Diet for a New America,* Tiburon, California: H. J. Kramer, 1987, p. 74.

18. Zambita, *Unadorned Thread of Yoga,* p. 31, translation adapted from Bailey.

19. http://news.nationalgeographic.com/news/2009/11/091123-thanksgiving-dinner-turkey-facts.html.

20. http://www.google.com/publicdata?ds=uspopulation&met=population&tdim=true&dl=en&hl=en&q=united+states+population.

BIBLIOGRAPHY

Gannon, Sharon, *Yoga and Vegetarianism*, San Rafael, California: Mandala Publishing, 2008.

Gannon, Sharon and David Life, *The Jivamukti Yoga Book*, New York: Ballantine Books, 2002.

Houston, Vyaas, *The Yoga Sutra Workbook: The Certainty of Freedom*: Warwick, New York: American Sanskrit Institute, 1995.

Lyman Howard and Glen Merzer, *Mad Cowboy: Plan Truth from the Cattle Rancher Who Won't Eat Meat*, New York: Scribner, 1998.

Mishra, Ramamurti S., *The Textbook of Yoga Psychology*, Monroe, New York: Baba Bhagavan Publication Trust, 1963.

Roach, Geshe Michael and Christie McNally, *The Essential Yoga Sutra*, New York: Three Leaves Press: 2005.

Robbins, John, *Diet For a New America*, Tiburon, California: H. J. Kramer Inc. 1987.

Scully, Matthew, *Dominion: The Power of Man, the Suffering of Animals and the Call to Mercy*, New York: St. Martin's Press, 2002.

Tuttle, Will, Ph.D., *The World Peace Diet: Eating for Spiritual Health and Social Harmony*, New York: Lantern Books, 2005.

Zambita, Salvatore, *The Unadorned Thread of Yoga: The Yoga Sutra of Patanjali in English*, a Compilation of English Translations of Sri Patanjali's Exposition of the Yoga Darshana, Poulsbo, Washington: The Yoga Sutras Institute Press, 1992.

7

Maharishi's Message: Vegetarianism as Natural Evolution

David P. Carter and Marguerite Regan

A young man raised his hand. "Is it alright to eat meat?"

A hush fell over the room. Maharishi Mahesh Yogi lowered his bearded chin and focused his eyes on the questioner. Then he lifted his forearm, pinched the flesh, and shook it with his hand. "We're made of meat, aren't we?" Eyes aglow, he burst into gales of laughter so rollicking that his whole frame shook with merriment.

The two dozen or so young American men and women who had gathered to hear him in a suite on the upper floor of New York's ritzy Plaza Hotel sat perplexed. Was Maharishi advocating vegetarianism? This is not an easy question to answer on the basis of his response. What are we to make of the ambiguity of it? It seems odd, especially given that Maharishi's spiritual lineage descended from the venerable Adi Shankaracharya, one of India's preeminent philosophers, a strict adherent of vegetarianism.[1] Not only was Shankaracharya vegetarian, so were his spiritual heirs.

Maybe Maharishi's ambiguous response was a ploy, a strategic welcome to both vegetarians and meat eaters. After all, it afforded both parties justification for their dietary practices. But ascribing tactical motives to the double entendre does not resolve the potent cognitive challenge it raises. What is its underlying, hidden meaning? On the one hand, "we're made of meat" could be an endorsement of flesh eating—following the line of reasoning that since we're made of meat, meat is the natural building block needed by the body to promote health and wellbeing. Consequently, we should eat meat; why even ask such a question? On the other hand, "we're made of meat" can just as easily be interpreted as an injunction against flesh eating. After all, as beings possessed of bodies made of meat, the answer begs a chilling question: how would *you* like to be eaten? Clearly, just as we do not want to be eaten, it stands to reason that neither do animals. Pursuing this line of reasoning further, we can unpack another denunciation of flesh eating from Maharishi's answer. Because human animals share bodily similarity with other animals—both possess bodies made of meat—a degree of kinship, however remote we may declare it to be, is there. Those who devour their kin are universally stigmatized. To feed on one's kin is unconscionable. It is cannibalism. His was a heavy answer, then—diplomatic, but heavy.

But could this really be what Maharishi meant when speaking to a group of American hippies one sunny afternoon in 1968? After all, his entire career reveals him as one who saw speaking and moralizing against meat eating as fruitless. Consequently, he required no special dietary standards for those trained to teach the Transcendental Meditation program or become leaders in his international society. In fact, aside from the regular daily practice of Transcendental Meditation (TM), little is asked of Maharishi's followers. To receive initiation into the practice, one simply has to abstain from intoxicants before instruction, and this period of abstinence varies in accordance with the substance in question. In order to achieve the desired result from regular practice, one also agrees to maintain subsequent sobriety. Maharishi also insisted that those trained by him as teachers must be well dressed at all times when in public and that, if men, they be clean shaven, with hair appropriately short and neatly trimmed to distinguish them from "hippies," an association he did not wish to encourage. Apart from sobriety and neat dress, that was it. There were no other strictures to observe, no set of religious beliefs to follow, no ritual practices, and no ethical or moral injunctions except to be law-abiding citizens of the state one lived in. There were no recommendations about recreation, cultural activities, movie going, sports events, or the like.

The key to unraveling Maharashi's stance on vegetarianism lies in adopting another approach to answering the question. "Example is better than precept," goes the old saw. Taking a cue from that wisdom, the riddle raised by Maharishi's equivocation is answered by his behavior. According to Fred Gratzon, Trustee of the Maharishi University of Management and longtime TM practitioner, Maharishi's diet was strictly lacto-vegetarian, and his attire was consistent with the nonviolence vegetarians endorse—he did not wear leather; his sandals were of wood and rubber.[2] And, although he sat on a deerskin, as is customary for Indian Yogis, the animal's pelt is traditionally obtained not as a byproduct of slaughter, but only after the animal's natural death.[3] Moreover, Gratzon reports that in all of the courses he attended since 1969, the food has been almost exclusively vegetarian (dairy—yes, eggs—no), with "one rare exception." In 1970, chicken and turkey were available at a course held in Estes Park, Colorado. Apart from that, Gratzon writes, "I am unaware of any other deviation."[4] Maharishi's own personal example, then, is supportive of vegetarianism.

There were his utterances as well, few and far between. According to Gratzon, Maharishi seldom talked about diet. If pressed, however, he might respond with a decidedly unambiguous statement supporting vegetarianism such as "I cannot imagine any sensible person eating dead animals" or "don't eat poison." While the latter statement might be cryptic for those unacquainted with Yogic tradition, it is not so for those familiar with Yoga's philosophy and praxis. Such persons can easily detect Maharishi's silent advocacy of vegetarianism. After all, Yogic discourse classifies all phenomena, food included, according to three distinct modes of nature: *sattva guna, raja guna, and tama guna*. It also articulates practical imperatives that derive from those classifications.

For example, *sattvic* foods such as leaves, flowers, stalks, roots, tubers, legumes, grains, fruits, berries, dairy products, nuts, and seeds are deemed suitable to the Yogic lifestyle; they are classified as fresh, wholesome, pure, creative, and uplifting, and are said to promote intelligence, strength, virtuous behavior, and longevity. On the other hand, *rajasic* foods such as garlic, onions, coffee, and tea are to be avoided as they are energizing in an unwholesome way that promotes unwelcome behavior and deterioration of health. Forbidden altogether are *tamasic* foods such as meat, fish, eggs, alcoholic beverages, and drugs, which are classified as dulling and parasitic. They subvert humanity's finer qualities such as compassion and morality, and are said to promote illness, inertia, and premature death. So, within the context of the Yogic tradition and lifestyle, this is what obtains when one unpacks Maharishi's statement "don't eat poison." And in this light, his meaning is entirely unambiguous.

Still, Maharishi did not openly or forcefully preach vegetarianism. For him, vegetarianism was a state of ethical living brought about not by didacticism and prescript but by contact with the transcendent. In his address to the 15th World Vegetarian Congress held in Madras, India, in 1957, he presented solutions to the "problem of safety of life, of love, protection, peace and happiness" for the whole of creation.[5] He agreed with the premise of the congress that vegetarianism was a direct means of protecting life on earth. But he did not think that vegetarianism could be established through didactic appeals. "Speaking does not go a long way to change a man," he argued. But he did not stop there:

> How are we going to change hardness and cruelty of heart to softness and overflowing love for everybody? Through platform speaking? No, it is not possible. Through outer suggestions? No, it is not possible. Through singing

the values of vegetarianism into the ears of the non-vegetarians? No, because their ears may receive the message, but the hardness of their heart will repel it.[6]

According to Maharishi, the only way to transform the spirit of killing, aggression, and violence into "the spirit of kindness and love ... for the whole creation" is for people to have direct experience of the blissful nature of the soul such that they become completely transformed. This experience, according to Maharishi, is available through the simple Transcendental Meditation technique.

My own transition to vegetarianism parallels Maharishi's recommendation that the adopting of vegetarianism be a natural evolution for a person and not the result of didactic speeches.[7] I first met Maharishi in 1968, and three years later, in October of 1971, I realized my dream of going abroad to study with him, not in Rishikesh, India, but in Mallorca, Spain. I was not alone—two thousand others had gathered for the teacher training, young people mostly from America and Europe. For the duration of the course each of us lived in a private room alone, even the married couples, as celibacy was enjoined on all to help establish one-pointed focus on our studies. Discipline was intense. Over the weeks and months of our studies, the practice of deep Transcendental Meditation was lengthened by daily increments until finally meditation became a round-the-clock immersion in transcendence. Each day Maharishi lectured on the philosophy of Yoga, and over time trained us how to teach others the art and science of transcendence.

As I remember it, breakfast and lunch were light, typically yogurt, fresh fruit, bread, and milk or fruit juice. As the course went on, though, we meditated more and ate less. In time, breakfast became a meal that was left outside of each meditator's door, with each meditator free to partake or forgo the offered items. If I am not misremembering, after a while, lunch disappeared from the daily routine as well. Supper, however, was different, especially in the beginning weeks. Each day, in groups of several hundred, meditators would dine in one or another of the large and well-appointed dining halls. The fare was delectable, mostly a variety of appetizing vegetables (it was there that I was first tasted Swiss chard) and mildly seasoned grains. Seafood was also an option, which suited me because over the three years I had followed Maharishi, I had fallen away from strict observance of vegetarianism and ate fish.

When I first met Maharishi, I was strict in my observance, but due to pressure from family and friends who convinced me that a strict vegetarian diet put my health at risk and could lead to irreparable damage, I relaxed my principles. By 1969, I had gone back to a diet that included fish, fowl, and eggs. Gradually, though, as I educated myself in the science of health and nutrition, I learned that the perils my family and friends had persuaded me of were ungrounded fears based on a lack of knowledge, and I began the slow return to a vegetarian diet. I had already largely recovered, having given up first fowl and then eggs. But, the evolution was incomplete. I persisted in eating fish.

One day during the teacher training in Mallorca, I decided to dine on shrimp. As usual, I sat conversing with my friends as we waited for our meals. But when the fateful platter arrived, one look at the shrimp altered me forever. From the otherwise innocent platter I saw staring back at me two dozen pairs of teeny, black eyes. And each of these dead bodies was equipped with two tight rows of once lively little legs (hairy seeming) which tapered into long, thin, claw-like feet. This made for a creepy, crawly sight that instantly took away my appetite. I sent the order back posthaste with the silent vow to never again dine on creatures plucked from their home in the sea to become a feast of dead bodies for my pleasure. It is a vow I have never regretted, never broken, and never once had difficulty keeping. No sermon or exhortation could have changed my heart as powerfully or completely as had the sight of those dead bodies piled one atop the other, the tangle of useless limbs, or the frightened, sightless eyes, pleading still though dead. My heart heard the mute cry of the voiceless dead: *shrimp are victims, seafood is carrion, meat is murder!*

Clearly, my own personal transformation followed the trajectory that Maharishi articulated in his address to the World Vegetarian Congress. Spiritual regeneration through meditation and not "platform speaking" is the only way to heal the world. The practice of Maharishi's Transcendental Meditation technique for years had been transforming my heart, and it was this transformed heart that viewed the dead creatures as just that, without the intervention of lusty appetite to blind me any longer. Maharishi knew that ultimately vegetarianism would be the result of regular practice. And, he knew that there were many like me, seekers of truth possessed of youthful energy and as yet unencumbered by the societal snares that overtake the older segments of the population, persons genuinely intent on adopting the Yogic lifestyle for the purpose of attaining spiritual enlightenment, but who were habituated by acculturation and circumstance to meat eating. He knew that words alone could not effect the necessary change. After all, he argued, for centuries advocates of reform had exhorted the masses to adopt ethical dietary habits, along with a host other evolutionary improvements, but to no avail: "All of the great religions of the world," he said, "have been speaking [against killing] from time immemorial—Eternal Vedas have been speaking of it, Holy Bible has been speaking of it, Holy Koran has been speaking of it, yet the killer kills."[8]

Rather than waste time on another doomed scheme, Maharishi proposed what he called the principle of the "second element." Unethical behavior is like darkness. Where there is darkness, he argued, attempting to deal with the darkness is futile. Because darkness is simply the absence of light, darkness cannot and will not be extirpated or stanched by any amount of manipulation or attack. Only by bringing light will the darkness be vanquished. Where light is, there can be no darkness, he taught. The light the world needed was the Transcendental Meditation technique he brought. This was his message. With this technique, the whole host of unethical practices, from animal slaughter to the amassing of genocidal weapons of mass destruction, would be dissipated, and an age of enlightenment would dawn.

Maharishi sought to bring the Transcendental Meditation technique to the world by establishing the Maharishi International University (MIU) in 1971. In 1974, MIU purchased and moved into the vacated campus of what was formerly Parsons College in Fairfield, Iowa. Along with teaching Transcendental Meditation and other courses, the fully accredited university (now called Maharishi University of Management) became "the first U.S. college to offer an organic, vegetarian, freshly prepared menu" on the grounds that it is healthier for both the individual and the environment.[9] Much of the food served in the campus dining hall is grown locally (in huge greenhouses during the winter). In fact, MUM boasts a Sustainability Living program that includes dairies, greenhouses, ecovillages, and an organic farm,[10] where, according to Gratzon, the plants even receive Vedic chanting. Milk comes from a local organic dairy that lets its cows retire to pasture (as opposed to being sent to the meat packer) when they no longer give milk—a practice that is extremely rare.

Moreover, the dairy farmer, Francis Thicke, even ran for Iowa's Secretary of Agriculture in November of 2010. Clearly, MUM is one of the more environmentally progressive colleges in North America, again the result not of a preachy environmentalism but a natural evolution based on meditation. Gratzon testifies to the environmental progressivism at MUM when he writes, "[A]ctivist folks . . . in Fairfield started (and are on the leading edge of) the opposition to genetically engineered food. Maharishi came out extremely strongly against GMOs many years ago. As a result, we here in Fairfield won't touch the stuff."[11]

There's no telling what became of those two dozen or so hippies who gathered in New York's Plaza Hotel back in 1968 to hear Maharishi speak or whether they took up meditation and vegetarianism. Certainly, times have changed. Maybe the filmmakers and wordsmiths of today who flood the world with dystopian and apocalyptic visions are well advised in their pessimism; maybe the Summer of Love was an anomaly that will never come again. But one thing is clear. After observing the evolution of those of our Yogic friends who have maintained their regular spiritual practices as outlined above, it is safe to say that one who applies the practices given by Maharishi evolves in spiritual consciousness to live an increasingly compassionate, joyous, and loving lifestyle. This lifestyle naturally includes vegetarianism.

NOTES

1. Though there are various traditions regarding Adi Shankaracharya's diet, it is commonly understood that he was an incarnation of Lord Shiva, who never partakes of nonvegetarian food. See http://www.hindudharmaforums.com/showthread.php?t=189.

2. Gratzon, Fred. Personal email correspondence. Aug. 30, 2010.

3. Ibid.

4. Ibid.

5. Address to the 15th World Vegetarian Congress 1957. International Vegetarian Union Website. http://www.ivu.org/congress/wvc57/maharishi.html.

6. Ibid., paras. 3–4.

7. In April of 1967, after searching for a qualified guru to guide him to enlightenment, coauthor David Carter accepted Maharishi Mahesh Yogi as his spiritual mentor and guide. In June of that same year, he was formally initiated into Maharishi's Transcendental Meditation (TM) system, and in October of 1971 he embarked on a course of study with Maharishi that culminated in his becoming a teacher of TM and the Science of Creative Intelligence (SCI) in June of 1972. He taught formal TM classes from 1972–1984 in various locations around New York City and the tri-state area. Over the years beginning in 1967, and on two separate continents, he received personal and private instruction from TM guides trained by Maharishi, from Maharishi himself, and from another distinguished Indian born *sadhu* associated with Maharishi, Brahmachary Satyanand.

8. Address to the 15th World Vegetarian Congress 1957, para. 3.

9. "Organic Vegetarian Meals." Maharishi University of Management Webpage. http://www.mum.edu/meals.html.

10. "Sustainability." Maharishi University of Management Webpage. http://www.mum.edu/sustainability.html.

11. Gratzon, op. cit.

Roots, Shoots, and *Ahimsa*: The Jain Yoga of Vegetarianism

Christopher Key Chapple

Jainism presents perhaps the oldest continuing practice of vegetarianism. The faith of Jainism arose in the centuries before the life of the Buddha, perhaps taking form in the eighth century BCE in the northeastern area of India. It continues in two primary denominations: the Svetamabara found largely in western India and the Digambara, found mainly in central and southern India, though adherents to each path can be found throughout India and throughout the world. One central teaching defines Jainism: nonviolence or *ahimsa*.

This chapter will trace the foundations for Jainism's nonviolent ethic by examining the principle of the "ensouledness" of all life forms as found in its earliest written literature, the *Acharanga Sutra*, circa 300 BCE. It will also explore Jain medieval biological treatises and modern teachings.

Jainism regards each life form (*jiva*) to be worthy of protection. The Jain tradition has set forth one of the earliest and most pervasive campaigns for vegetarianism in global history. Along with Buddhism, it severely criticized the Brahmanical practice of animal sacrifice as violent and wasteful. Copious literature codifies the Jain definition of life. Various Jain texts on karma delineate consequences that arise due to violence committed against animals. Jain historical figures advocated successfully for limited animal protection under the Mughal rule. Even today, the Jains continue to adapt their interpretations of how best to observe nonviolence, resulting in the recent advocacy of veganism by members of the Jain diaspora.

THE JAIN WORLDVIEW

Jain cosmology posits a complex universe in the shape of a human body. In the lower realms of seven hells, individuals who were once people suffer due to heinous deeds committed in past lives. In the middle zone, also known as Jambudvipa, multiple life forms abound. Situated on continents divided by oceans and punctuated with rivers, this earthly realm includes various modalities (*gatis*) into which the soul (*jiva*) is born. These births include elemental bodies of earth, water, fire, and air, in which one may dwell as a rock, a drop of dew, a flame, or as the life within a gust of wind; microorganisms and plants; and insects, fish, reptiles, amphibians, and animals, including human beings. If a person is particularly virtuous, that person may ascend to one of nine heavens, experiencing great pleasure and even power.

Eventually, however, even the gods and goddesses must descend, as their pleasures are only temporary. Depending upon one's actions (*karma*), a soul will return into a new body after death for round after round of birth and rebirth. In the Jain system, each soul is unique and contains an energy and movement that propels it forward repeatedly until one takes an interest in and makes a commitment to reversing the karmas that condemn a person to the cycle of life, death, and rebirth. Such an individual has the opportunity, through his or her own effort, to expunge all the influences of karma and ascend to the limits of the universe, beyond all material entrapments, dwelling forevermore in a state of perfect knowledge and bliss.

The Jain path to freedom requires one deceivingly simple practice: the cultivation of nonviolence in thought, word, and deed. The knots of karma bind up a soul into a colorful package that must be carefully unwrapped. Every act of violence, however subtle, thickens the glue of obscuring karma. To undo the knots and melt the glue, one must develop vigilance at the practice of five vows designed to release the soul from its bondage. These five, which were also taken up by Patanjali as the core ethical principles for Yoga, are nonviolence, truthfulness, nonstealing, sexual restraint, and nonpossessiveness.[1] The cultivation of the first, nonviolence, has resulted in a distinct lifestyle for the Jain community that includes an ongoing commitment to vegetarianism.

JAINISM AND YOGA

Threads of Jainism can be detected in Patanjali's Yoga. In Patanjali's eightfold path, the ethical practices of nonviolence, truthfulness, not stealing, sexual restraint, and nonpossession (*Yoga Sutra* 2:29–39), are identical with the vows listed in the *Acaranga Sutra*, as noted above. The description of karma as black, white, or mixed (*Yoga Sutra* 4:7) corresponds with the more detailed description of the range of colors (black, blue, red, yellow, white) in Jain texts (see *Tattvartha Sutra* 5:24 and 9:49). The culmination of Yoga in the state known as perfect aloneness (*kaivalyam*) as described in Patanjali (*Yoga Sutra* 2:25; 3:50, 55; 4:26, 34) bears close similarity to the Jain articulation of freedom (*kevala*, as in *Tattvartha Sutra*, 1:9, 1:30, 10:4).

Patanjali defines Yoga as "*chitta vritti nirodha*," the restraint of mental fluctuations. Other authors equate Yoga with a state of union with the divine. The Jains use the word Yoga in a general sense to refer to all things that lead one into the path of *Dharma*, in the sense of all-purpose spirituality. A "Yogi" in Jain literature refers to an accomplished monk, capable of teaching and inspiring others in the Jain faith. However, the Jains also use the word Yoga in a technical sense to refer to the process by which karma binds itself to the soul, impeding its spiritual journey. The Jains outline a 14-fold path of stages (*gunasthanas*) through which one ascends to the point of total freedom. The penultimate step is referred to as *Yoga Kevala*, indicating that one still possesses the karmas necessary to abide within the human form. At the final step, *Ayoga Kevala*, one releases or disassociates or unlinks oneself from the final remnants of karma, attaining eternal energy, consciousness, and bliss. This distinction is not unlike Bhojaraja's preference to refer to *viyoga* or separation of soul (*purusha*) from manifest reality (*prakriti*) as the culmination of Yoga.

For the purposes of this chapter, let it be known that both Patanjali and Mahavira (the Jain Master) agree upon the need for a particular practice of Yoga: the observance of *ahimsa*, the precept of nonviolence. Both traditions emphasize that adherence to nonviolence is central to spiritual practice and cannot be negotiated. Patanjali proclaims that its practice must not be limited by "birth, place, time, or circumstance at all times" (*Yoga Sutra* 2:31) and that its perfection results in "the abandonment of all hostility in one's presence" (*Yoga Sutra* II:35). The most visible form of nonviolent practice can be seen in vegetarianism, perfected and promulgated in the Jain tradition as explained below.

VEGETARIAN ORIGINS

The earliest surviving text of the Jain tradition, the *Acharanga Sutra*, dates from the third century BCE. It sets forth a strong and uncompromising message: do not harm animals. The text establishes the various uses that one can make of animals and then unequivocally condemns anyone who commits those acts and causes or allows others to do so:

Some slay animals for sacrificial purposes, some kill animals for the sake of their skin, some kill them for the sake of their flesh, some kill them for the sake of their blood; thus for the sake of their heart, their bile, the feathers in their tale, their tail, their big or small horns, their teeth, their tusks, their nails, their sinews, their bones; with a purpose or without a purpose. Some kill animals because they have been wounded by them, or are wounded, or will be wounded.

The one who injures these animals does not comprehend and renounce the sinful acts; the one who does not injure these animals comprehends and renounces the sinful acts. A wise person should not act sinfully toward animals, or cause others to do so, nor should they allow others to behave in this way.[2]

The author goes on to state that "All beings are fond of life, like pleasure, hate pain, shun destruction, like life, long to live. To all, life is dear"[3] and "One should not kill, nor cause others to kill, nor consent to the killing of others."[4] Thus, the protection of all life is key to the Jain path. By killing, one increases one's karma, defined as the root cause of all suffering. Hence, "all breathing, existing, living, sentient creatures should not be slain, nor treated with violence, nor abused, nor tormented, nor driven away. This is the pure, unchangeable, eternal law."[5]

The observant Jain heeds the advice of the *Acharanga Sutra* given as follows:

Knowing and renouncing severally and singly the actions against living beings, in the regions above, below, and on the surface, everywhere and in all ways, a wise person neither gives pain to these bodies, nor orders others to do so, nor assents to their doing so. We abhor those who give pain to these bodies. Knowing this, a wise person should not cause this or any other pain to any beings.[6]

These teachings were formulated and expressed by Mahavira Vardhamana, also known as "the Jina," who lived around the fifth century BCE, a contemporary of the Buddha. Regarded to be the most recent great teacher, or *tirthankara*, in a line of 24 founders of the faith, his life serves as a paradigm for observant Jains. Hailing from a princely family, he renounced worldly life at the age of 30, wandered for 12 years, achieved the blessed state of freedom (*kevala*) and then taught for 40 years before embarking on his final act of nonviolence, the renunciation of all food until death. The *Acharanga Sutra* describes the monastic diet that sustained Mahavira during his years of wandering: "rice, pounded jujube, and beans."[7] It also outlines a practice of regular fasting, wherein Mahavira is said to have eaten only every 6th, 8th, 10th, or 12th meal.

For Jain monks and nuns who follow Mahavira's teachings, not only must the food be strictly vegetarian, they must be careful to make certain that no "eggs, nor living beings . . . nor ants . . . nor cobwebs" contaminate their food.[8] It is noted that "If a monk or nun would eat or drink without inspecting the food and drink, he or she might hurt and displace or injure or kill all sorts of living beings.[9] They are also strictly prohibited from accepting alcohol or the juice of the following fruits if they have begun to ferment: "mangos, apples, citrons, grapes, dates, pomegranates, cocoanuts, bamboos, jujubes, myrobalans, and tamarinds."[10] Numerous rules are given about the fruits and vegetables that are deemed acceptable to eat, and the conditions in which they are prepared.

Jain monks and nuns (*sadhus* and *sadhvis*) are also encouraged to develop a friendly view toward animals:

> A monk or nun, seeing a man, a cow, a buffalo, deer, cattle, a bird, a snake, an aquatic animal of increased bulk, should not speak about them in this way: "He (or it) is fit, round, fit to be killed or cooked;" considering well, they should not use such [language, which is] sinful, blamable, rough, stinging, coarse, hard, leading to sins, to discords and factions, to grief and outrage, to destruction of living beings.[11]

Instead, monks and nuns are encouraged to celebrate the beauty of animals, to praise them for their dignity rather than see them as objects to be consumed or manipulated.

THE BIOLOGICAL VIEW

Animals are arranged according to an interesting hierarchy of life in the *Tattvartha Sutra*, the classical text that outlines Jain cosmology, composed by Umasvati most likely in the fifth century of the CE. This terse text delineates the nature of the soul (*jiva*), specifying particular types of karmas that adhere to and hence occlude the inherent radiance of the soul, binding her to further rebirth. Souls according to Jainism are eternal and are constantly taking on new shapes and forms up until the point of final liberation from karma, after which no further rebirth occurs. Souls are found in the elements of earth, water, fire, and air, as well as in microbes and plants, all of which are said to have the sense of touch through which they manifest consciousness. As life forms become more complex, they add senses: worms add taste, bugs add smell, flying insects add sight; fish and reptiles add hearing. This hierarchy culminates with mammals, who think in addition to having the capacity to touch, taste, smell, and see. Umasvati writes:

The worldly souls fall into two groups,
souls that possess a mind and souls that do not.
The worldly souls are further classified as mobile and immobile beings.
The earth-bodied, water-bodied and plant-bodied souls are immobile beings.
Fire and air, as well as those with two or more senses, are mobile beings.[12]

The commentaries on the *Tattvartha Sutra* specify the life span of various forms of life and delineate the various forms of birth that give rise to life, from the spontaneous arising of plants from seeds to uterine and egg-hatching forms of birth. Each of these forms of life arises due to configurations of karma, described in Jainism as sticky, colorful, and mobile. Each soul has volition that attracts particular particles of karma, resulting in rebirth and suffering due to instincts rooted in hunger, fear, lust, and greed.[13] One observes vegetarianism in order to avoid attracting these negative karmas that will obscure the soul.

Jain author Hemacandra (1089–1172) created a list of forbidden (*abhaksya*) foods. These include the fruits of five forms of fig (*umbara, vata, pippala, plaksa, kakombari*); the four foods and liquids to be universally avoided (the meat of birds, reptiles, fish, or mammals; alcohol; honey; and butter); plants with bulbs or rhizomes including potatoes, carrots, onions, and garlic; fruits with many seeds; food eaten at night; pulses with raw milk products; fermented rice; curd more than two days old; and tainted food.[14]

John Cort notes that "Actual dietary practice varies widely from individual to individual and from household to household, and overlaps only in part with the *abhaksyas*. . . . In this it differs to some extent from lists of prohibited foods found in the Jewish and Muslim traditions."[15] In my own experience, many modern urban Jains both in India and in the United States will eat at night in a brightly lit room. They will carefully avoid ordering eggplant when dining out and will be scrupulous in presenting "proper" vegetarian fare when entertaining at home. Many modern Jains will eat root vegetables, though this is rarely the case among elders. Due to the teaching that action performed in the last third of one's life will predetermine the nature of one's next birth, many Jains over 50 become more abstemious and observant, fasting more frequently, and being careful, in some instances, not to eat foods that would have been acceptable when they were younger.

VEGETARIAN PRACTICES

One distinctive aspect of Jain vegetarianism is the unique view taken of vegetables, which are divided into two groups. One group contains just one soul, while the other group harbors countless souls. This latter group includes several root vegetables that are not consumed by observant Jains: potatoes, carrots, onions, garlic, and yams.[16] Some Jains proclaim that the reason that they avoid root vegetables is that many life forms are disturbed and harmed when the plant is pulled from the ground.[17] Another variant of vegetarianism among Jains is to forego leafy green vegetables during the rainy season, when they are likely to harbor insects[18] and on certain days in the lunar month known as *tithi*. It is important for observant Jains to avoid fruits or vegetables that have a large number of seeds, such as tomatoes or eggplant.

In addition to consuming only vegetarian food, traditional Jains also eschew eating after sunset to avoid eating insects that one cannot see due to darkness. Cort interviewed a Jain monk who commented, "After sunset many subtle and minute living beings are bred . . . and so are killed when they are eaten. Eating at night causes indigestion and harms our health. We feel indolent. . . . By eating at night, we may die from eating poisonous creatures which come into the food." The monk asserts that night eating can cause cancer, dropsy, vomiting, fever, and death.[19]

Another practice related to eating shows the care put forward in regard to even microscopic life. In order to prevent the needless proliferation of life, it is important not to take more food than one can finish. Waste will generate countless beings that will die a painful death, a death that would be avoidable by not taking more than one can consume. These beings are seen not only as bacteria (*nigoda*) but also as arising from an individual's saliva and hence producing a miniature version of one's own being. As noted by Babb, "some ascetics and extra-orthodox laymen drink the liquid residue from washing their hands and plates or bowls. This is to prevent the spontaneous generation of millions of little replicas of themselves, for whose deaths they would then be responsible, in the meal's remains."[20] Additionally, to avoid the harm that goes into the production of food, Jain monks and nuns are not allowed to prepare food for themselves, but must receive it from lay devotees.

The Jain faith has developed an extraordinary variety of fasts (*upvas*) that serve as occasions to refrain from taking all forms of life, thus purifying oneself of harmful karmas. These fasts can be for one day up to 45 days and can be selective in terms of foods avoided and liquids allowed. Many fasts last for three days or eight meals. The most rigorous fasts allow only water. During the *ambil* fast, generally practiced once or twice each month, one takes only rice, gruel, or barley meal. The most well-known community fast, *paryushan*, takes place in late August or early September, during which all Jains attempt to purify themselves through food restriction for a full week.[21] As can be deduced, not only must the desire for nonvegetarian food be renounced, ultimately, desire for all food must dissipate in order to advance the soul to freedom. Padmanabh S. Jaini states that "The path of *moksha* consists in overcoming the desire for food in all its forms, for true liberation is freedom from hunger forever."[22] Four cravings lie at the heart of human existence: food, fear, sex, and possessions. All must be abandoned for an individual to achieve freedom. By observing the Jain vows, one gradually erodes the influence of karmic cravings; vegetarianism is a critical piece of this process.

ADVOCACY OF VEGETARIANISM

From before the time of the Buddha, Jains have advocated vegetarianism. They have tirelessly introduced legislation for animal protection and have opened and maintained thousands of animal shelters all throughout India.[23] One of the most famous instances of vegetarian advocacy occurred under Mughal rule. A Jain leader, the Dadaguru Jincandrasuri (1541–1613), according to one account convinced the Mugha Emperor Akbar to forbid the slaughter of animals for one week per year, in honor of the Jain faith,[24] while other accounts extend the ban on animal slaughter to six months per year and even claim that Akbar personally renounced hunting. Another Jain teacher from this period, Hiravijaya Suri (1527–95), reportedly convinced Akbar to "issue decrees ordering the freeing of caged birds and the banning of the slaughter of animals on the Svetamabara festival of Paryushan."[25] His pupil Shanticandra continued to advocate Jain and vegetarian causes at the court.

A contemporary Jain religious leader, Acharya Mahaprajna endorses vegetarianism for some of the following reasons:

> Nonvegetarians suffer from an excessive intake of protein. Moreover, it too is an established fact that animal protein is not as useful as vegetable protein. For examples, millet protein is good for health while meat protein causes disease. Not only this, a non-vegetarian has to use alcohol and/or excessive salt to digest meat, which causes diseases of the kidneys, liver and heart. To quite some extent food is responsible for some of the major killer diseases like hypertension, cardiac troubles, ulcers, cancer, and kidney failure. . . . Most emotional disturbances in modern society can be blamed on the use of intoxicants and non-vegetarian food.[26]

Today, Jains continue to campaign for vegetarianism and protection of animals with traveling exhibitions and billboards[27] in India and by promoting and supporting animal shelters in India and abroad.

VEGANISM

Pravin K. Shah of Carey, North Carolina, published an essay that has been widely circulated on the Internet, "My Visit to a Dairy Farm." In this first-person account he describes modern dairy practices and his consequent repugnance toward dairy products. Milk and milk products have long been a staple of the Jain diet, with the exception of cheeses hardened by animal rennet. Prior to Shah's investigative reporting, most Jains would not have given a second thought to drinking milk or eating yogurt or cottage cheese. However, this essay, which has been circulated in various forms, and Shah's untiring presence at various Jain community gatherings, have begun a movement within Jainism toward becoming vegan, relying only on plant-food sources, and abandoning dairy products.

Shah's shock can be gleaned from the following passages that document his visit to a dairy farm in Vermont in May, 1995:

> [T]he machine was milking the cow . . . without regard to how hard it was on the cow. It was extremely difficult for me to watch the cows' sufferings during the milking. To extract the last drop of milk, sometimes traces of blood got mixed with the milk. . . . The evening I was there, the farm was shipping three baby calves in a truck to a veal factory. The mother cows were crying when their babies were separated from them. . . . The veal industry is the most cruel meat industry in the world. . . . The baby calves are raised in the darkness in a very confining crate, which allows practically no movements, and are fed an iron-deficient diet. . . . About four to five times a year, this farm would take the cows outside for a walk. Otherwise, the cows are tied in one place and they have no choice but to defecate where they are confined.

This experience moved Shah to take up veganism, though not without an internal struggle:

> How could I eliminate milk, yogurt, butter, ghee, and cheese from my diet? . . . I cannot drink tea, eat any Indian sweets, pizza, milk chocolate, [or] ice cream. However, needless to say that the dairy farm tour made me an instant vegan. I was 55 years old when I became vegan. . . . My doctor is very pleased with my results. . . . Cholesterol [went from] 205 [to] 160; HDL [went from] 34 [to] 42; Triglycerides [went from] 350 [to] 175. . . .

Though Shah attests to the health benefits of veganism, his major concern is the well-being of the cow:

> The cow is a five-sensed (Panchendriya) animal and cruelty to a Panchendriya animal is considered the highest sin and is totally prohibited even by

the Jain lay people.... [D]uring milk production the cows are not killed instantly but they are tortured badly during their prime life and ultimately slaughtered before the end of their natural life. The dairy cows have no chance to escape from this cruelty.[28]

Like many nonresident Indians, Shah had pleasant memories of cow treatment in India. These were dashed as he discovered that modern agricultural practices have become global, and that animals that once wandered free in India now endure long periods of confinement in unsanitary conditions. Shah goes on to suggest that Jains should not only stop using milk as a food source but also eliminate its extensive ritual use. Vast quantities of milk are used each day to bathe Jina images worldwide. Given the squalid conditions in which milk cows live, he suggests that their suffering would invalidate the efficacy of the ritual.

Each October, the 67 Jain centers in North America celebrate Gandhi Day through activities and programs that include disseminating information to the general public about the benefits of vegetarianism. Support networks within the Jain diaspora community encourage adherence to Jain dietary principles. Jain youth are educated about the benefits of vegetarianism through well-organized "Sunday schools" or *pathshalas* that inculcate Jain values, particularly the observance of vegetarianism.[29] The Federation of Jain Associations in North America has entered a partnership with the Physicians Committee for Responsible Medicine to encourage national standards that include vegetarian school lunches. They launched a joint grassroots lobbying campaign in April, 2010, in support of federal legislation, H.R. 4870, the Healthy School Meals Act.[30] As the Jain lay community prospers worldwide, it continues its long tradition, dating back more than 2,500 years, of urging others to respect and support and even adopt a vegetarian diet.

CONCLUSION

The Jain faith envisions the world as peopled with countless souls, continually taking new births according to their actions. Humans stand in the privileged position of having the capacity to understand the consequences of karma. Consequently, humans can decide to listen, to act upon a higher moral calling. Any act of violence further obscures the soul on its quest for freedom. Vegetarianism provides an avenue to reduce the binding, negative effects of karma on the soul. As a key aspect of the Jain code of conduct, vegetarianism allows one to reduce the direct and indirect harm caused by the consumption of flesh foods. As noted by Vilas Sangave, "though violence (*himsa*) is unavoidable in the sustenance of life, Jainism, by rules of conduct, tries to limit it for essential purposes only."[31]

Vegetarianism has distinguished the Jain community since its inception. The attention to detail given to different types of food, times when food should and not be consumed, and the elaborate rituals associated with fasting, are without parallel. Furthermore, the Jain community for centuries has advocated widespread adoption of vegetarianism, influencing Buddhists, Hindus, and more recently Christians, Jews, and modern secular individuals. Although the unique and compelling worldview that supports Jain vegetarianism might be at odds with the current wisdom of scientific cosmology, contemporary western medical research does in fact give credence to some of its claims that a vegetarian lifestyle helps improve the quality and longevity of human life. The Jain precept of nonviolence, rooted in a philosophy that sees and respects life in all places, sets vegetarianism at the core of Jain faith and practice.

NOTES

1. For more on the relationship between classical Yoga and Jainism, see Christopher Key Chapple, *Yoga and the Luminous: Patanjali's Spiritual Path to Freedom* (Albany: State University of New York Press, 2008) and *Reconciling Yogas: Haribhadra's Collection of Views on Yoga* (Albany: State University of New York Press, 2003).

2. *Acharanga Sutra* 1:1:5–6, in Hermann Jacobi, tr., *Jaina Sutras: Part One: Akaranga Sutra, Kalpa Sutra* (New York: Dover, 1968, first published at Clarendom Press, Oxford, 1884), p. 12. Abbreviated hereafter as AS.

3. AS I:2:3, Jacobi 19.

4. AS I:3:2, Jacobi 31.

5. AS IV:1:1, Jacobi 36.

6. AS I:7:2, Jacobi 63–64.

7. AS I:8:4, Jacobi 86.

8. AS II:1:1, Jacobi 8.

9. AS II:15:ii, Jacobi 204.

10. AS II:1:8, Jacobi 108.

11. AS II:4:2, Jacobi 153–154.

12. Nathmal Tatia, tr., *That Which Is: Tattvartha Sutra, A Classic Jain Manual for Understanding the True Nature of Reality* (San Francisco: HarperCollins, 1994), pp. 40–42.

13. Padmanabh S. Jaini, *Collected Papers on Jaina Studies* (Delhi: Motilal Banarsidass, 2000), p. 293.

14. R. Williams, *Jaina Yoga: A Survey of the Mediaeval Sravakacras* (Delhi: Motilal Banarsidass, 1983; first edition, Oxford, 1963), p. 110.

15. John E. Cort, *Jains in the World: Religious Values and Ideology in India* (Oxford: Oxford University Press, 2001), p. 128.

16. Lawrence A. Babb, *Absent Lord: Ascetics and Kings in a Jain Ritual Culture* (Berkeley: University of California Press, 1996), p. 45.

17. Josephine Reynell, "Women and the Reproduction of the Jain Community," in Michael Carrithers and Caroline Humphrey, *The Assembly of Listeners: Jains in Society* (Cambridge: Cambridge University Press, 1991), p. 55.

18. Marcus Banks, *Organizing Jainism in India and England* (Oxford: Clarendon Press, 1992), p. 18.

19. Cort, op. cit., p. 130.

20. Babb, op. cit., pp. 46–47.

21. Cort, op. cit., pp. 134–138.

22. Padmanabh S. Jaini, *Collected Papers on Jaina Studies* (Delhi: Motilal Banarsidass, 2000), p. 294.

23. See Deryck O. Lodrick, *Sacred Cows, Sacred Places: Origins and Survival of Animal Homes in India* (Berkeley: University of California Press, 1981).

24. Babb, op. cit., p. 124.

25. Paul Dundas, *The Jains* (London: Routledge, 1992), p. 126.

26. Yuvacharya Mahapragya, *Nonviolence and Its Many Aspects*, Second Edition, translated by R. P. Bhattnagar (Ladnun: Jain Vishva Bharati), p. 15.

27. James Laidlaw, *Riches and Renunciation: Religion, Economy, and Society among the Jains* (Oxford: Oxford University Press, 1995), p. 94.

28. Pravin K. Shah, "My Visit to a Dairy Farm," Worldwide Web, accessed April 28, 2010).

29. See www.jainpathshala.org, www.jaincenter.net, and www.jcgp.org/pathshala.

30. See www.jaina.org.

31. Vilas Sangave, *Jaina Religion and Community* (Long Beach, CA: Long Beach Publications, 1997), p. 168.

9

Bhakti-Yoga: Reflections on the Spirituality of Eating

Joshua M. Greene

A friend who is also a much-loved teacher of Bhakti-Yoga, the Yoga of devotion, told me about the day he became vegetarian. In 1970, at age 20, Richard Slavin traveled overland from Amsterdam to India seeking God. He survived a number of dangerous encounters before arriving in Delhi exhausted, starving, and broke. Within hours, hucksters had plied him with intoxicants, tied him up with a boa constrictor, and tricked him into eating fiery-hot peppers.

As evening approached, the boa came off and the effects of the drugs and peppers subsided. Richard had few belongings and no idea where to go. Standing in the street wondering what to do, he was approached by a gentleman who seemed curious to find a young Westerner on his own in India. The man invited Richard to dine with him at an outdoor restaurant. Their table was just inches from the road. The man ordered two meals, and as they sat waiting a white cow strolled by nuzzling her calf and lay down just next to their table. Richard had never been so close to a cow and he marveled at her graceful movements and big brown eyes. The cow doted on her calf, and Richard was struck by how closely the exchange resembled that of a human mother and her child.

A waiter rushed up and slapped down two plates. Richard had barely eaten in days and he delved into the food. Halfway through the meal his host asked, "Mr. Richard, would you like me to explain what all this is?" Pointing to each item he described, "This is *chaval*, or rice. This thing that looks like wheat bread is called *roti*. These vegetables are called *subji*. This soup over here is made with lentils, and we call it *dhal*. Here is a condiment or *chutney*." Then he pointed to some small chunks on the rice: "And this is meat."

Just then the cow leaned over to lick Richard's leg. Richard stared first at the meat, then at the cow, and realized with horror that all his life he had been an unwitting participant in a cruel and heartless practice. How could he be so insensitive to the suffering of an innocent child of God? Thinking of the millions of animals killed every day to be butchered and served up as someone's dinner he lost his composure and dissolved into tears. His host had no idea what was happening.

"Is something wrong, sir? Why are you so disturbed?"

Richard could barely speak. "Thank you for everything," he said standing up and pushing back his chair. "Please excuse me," he said. "I'm feeling ill." On his way out, he patted the cow, and the cow reciprocated by licking his hand.

Today Richard is known by his Bhakti name Radhanath Swami. "Before that moment," he told me, "I never made the connection between what I ate and my search for God. I just never saw it." His journey to God had begun long before that day, but realizing that "an innocent child of God" could live in a cow's body helped define where he was going. Becoming vegetarian had less to do with philosophy and health than realizing he had a relationship with all creatures big and small.

SPIRITUAL INTERCONNECTEDNESS

Someday, looking back from whatever post-apocalyptic future humanity is preparing, people may conclude that this generation's greatest failure was undervaluing relationships with life in its many breathtaking forms. What is exploitation of nature if not denial of our relationship with the Earth? What is animal slaughter if not a failure to honor our relationship with other species? To be sure, there are relative merits to vegetarianism on its own terms. We can eat healthier, cause less environmental damage, and reduce violence by giving up meat. But helpful as these changes would be, meat is the narrow wedge of a much larger dilemma: namely, our neglect of relationships as the foundation of progressive human culture. If we objectify animals as biological phenomena and deny our shared spiritual heritage, what stops us from doing the same with women, gays, Muslims, Jews, or any group from which we choose to differentiate ourselves? Another friend, a Bhakti-Yoga instructor at Columbia, communicates this idea to students by holding up two photos: one of a dog on a leash, the other of a cow being led to the killing floor of a slaughterhouse. Isn't it strange, he asks his students, that a dog-owner can be fined for keeping his pet on too short a leash, yet there are no consequences for butchering an innocent cow? We don't usually make that kind of connection for one simple reason: we have a relationship with our pets and understand our obligation to treat them humanely. No such relationship governs our treatment of cattle.

Recognizing that we are in a reciprocal relationship with all living beings defines Bhakti-Yoga. *Bhakti* texts say that bodies—human, animal, plant or otherwise—function as housing for eternal souls. Souls emanate from God and possess God's divine nature: eternity, knowledge, and bliss. Without the presence of this *atma* or spark of the Divine, a body cannot grow or move. The Sanskrit texts say that the *atma* is infinitely small yet extraordinarily powerful, metaphorically equivalent to ten thousand suns illuminating the universe of the body. Advancement in Bhakti-Yoga equals a practitioner's ability to honor this divine spark in whatever corporeal housing it may exist.

Acknowledging a relationship with other living beings means accepting that sometimes we cannot avoid causing them harm. Frequently people ask about pain caused to plants in a vegetarian diet. Doesn't harvesting plant life also constitute an abuse of other living beings? Among the many rationales I have heard, two strike me as worth repeating. The first is that plants do not have central nervous systems, and although they react to external stimuli, vegetables do not experience pain to the degree that vertebrate animals do. More important, the active principle in Bhakti-Yoga is not vegetarianism but devotion. In purchasing ingredients, practitioners are conscious of fruits, vegetables and the earth itself as manifestations of God. When considering what to buy, conscientious Bhakti-Yogis read labels and separate environmentally friendly companies from those that abuse nature. When possible, they avoid plastic and other contaminants. Beyond general proscriptions against harm, *Bhakti* elevates nonviolence to specific initiatives to minimize whatever damage our own needs might inflict on any life form. The Sanskrit phrase for such thinking is *para-duhkha-duhkhi*—"feeling the suffering of others"—not just the suffering of our own species but of all living beings.

None of this is new: there are devotional perspectives to diet in most traditional cultures. Buddhists call it the Buddha nature or the ability to empathize with suffering anywhere in the world. Native Americans, while not vegetarian, offer prayers to their prey and ask forgiveness for using them as food. Coastal peoples such as the Inuits chant hymns to fish and to the ocean. Of course, hunting the food they eat puts these groups into close contact with nature and favors awareness of relationships. Urban life estranges us from nature and devalues the connection between ourselves and other species. Purchasing industrially slaughtered, pre-packaged meat in supermarkets makes living beings seem like another commodity. Bhakti reforms that impression by reminding us that what we consume has divine origins. "A true Yogi," says Krishna, speaker of the Bhagavad Gita (BG), "sees me in all beings and sees all beings in me. Indeed, the self-realized person sees me everywhere" (BG 6.29).

In the beginning of devotional life, practitioners may become vegetarian because a nonmeat diet is healthy, economical, and environmentally friendly. More advanced Bhakti-Yogis have a different purpose. Beyond their own interests they ask, "What will please my Beloved?" That sentiment guides all their decisions. My point of reference for that kind of devotional thinking is my teacher, A. C. Bhaktivedanta Swami Prabhupada, who left India by boat in the summer of 1965, reaching America's shores one month later. A few years before his passing in 1977 I asked him about what a lover of God sees when looking at a tree. It was not the first time I had asked something presumptuous, but as usual he took it gracefully.

"A lover of God looks at a tree the way a mother looks at her child's shoes," he said. "She does not see just a shoe. She is thinking, 'This is my child's shoe.' She sees her child in that shoe because love is there. Similarly, a lover of God does not exactly see a tree. He thinks, 'Here is a soul inhabiting this tree body.' And what is that soul? Part and parcel of Krishna or God. So he is seeing the tree but thinking 'Krishna' because love is there." What a wonderful description of Yoga as a redefining of relationships.

SEEING GOD IN FOOD

There was a cook I knew who epitomized this mood of devotion. During my early days as a student at the London Radha Krishna Temple in 1969, I helped him prepare lunch for 30 temple residents. The cook's initiated name was Digvijaya. He was a short, round-faced Brit in his late twenties with a soft voice and a constant smile. Before starting to cook he would shower, anoint his body with clay markings in 12 places, as is the custom among Krishna devotees, and dress in clean clothes. We would meet in the kitchen around noon and while I washed and trimmed vegetables, he measured out cups of rice and carefully mixed precise amounts of turmeric, cumin, coriander, and other spices in wide pans of clarified butter called *ghee*. Digvijaya had been preparing three meals a day for the past two years and had developed a culinary choreography: he moved like a dancer through the kitchen, waltzing lightly around the room singing Bengali prayers while pulling down pots, rolling dough, and mixing vats of split-pea *dahl* soup, fruit drinks, and salad fixings. Soon the air was filled with the crackling of spice pods and a heady blend of sweet and pungent aromas.

When the foods were ready, Digvijaya ladled an individual portion of each into stainless steel bowls and arranged the bowls on a wide brightly polished tray. Over the vegetables he sprinkled a few leaves from the sacred Tulsi bush that grew by the kitchen window. To the tray he added a freshly cut flower, a cup of water, silverware and neatly pressed linen napkin. Then I helped him carry the heavy tray upstairs to the temple room and place it on the altar.

Ancient Sanskrit texts abound with stories attesting to the mystical qualities of *prasadam*, or "mercy," meaning foods that have been sanctified with prayers of offering to God. Lives have been saved, wars ended, darkness turned to light by a single grain of *prasadam* rice. Sage Narada, to cite a popular example, was orphaned at an early age and left without resources or support. Adopted by a group of hermit Bhaktas living in a forest, he shared their daily *prasadam* meals. Later in life, he credited this *prasadam* diet with his emergence as one of India's most influential philosopher-saints. In another popular story, Krishna ate one grain of rice from a dish offered to him with love, and the satisfaction he felt from that one grain was transferred to an entire army who then abandoned their plans for war.

Traditionally, *prasadam* is always vegetarian, for food offered to Krishna in sacrifice must consist of edibles of which he approves. Sacred texts make it abundantly clear: Krishna will not partake of foods that involve killing animals, and, therefore, neither will his devotees. Ultimately, however, transformation of food from common to sacred takes place in the heart, a sensation I first experienced during those early days in London. Once the tray had been positioned on the altar, Digvijaya and I would bow to the deities and offer prayers. The mental exercise during offering consists of humility. No matter how much we may have labored to prepare the meal, during the offering we sought no credit. Our tiny creation paled before the transcending majesty of nature that supplied the ingredients. Prayers of offering were our attempt to recognize God's role as the primal source of the elements from which each of us builds his or her life. The whole process of sanctifying food boils down to this effort at expressing gratefulness. Like that of an artist, the Bhakti-Yogi's role is to serve as conduit for returning the bounty of nature to its source.

After prayers, Digvijaya and I returned to the kitchen to serve lunch to our many guests. Residents and guests sat on cushions in two lines. We rolled large pots of rice, *dahl* soup, vegetables, and other *prasadam* down the lines on two dollies, spooning out portions and looking up at each guest: a little shake of head or wave of the hand meant "Thank you, that's plenty." Inevitably, everyone asked for second and third helpings and by the end guests were in awe over the tasty meal. The effect of these meals, especially on newcomers, was astonishing. Some would literally squeal with delight. Inevitably people laughed, as it seemed impossible that a meal could taste so good or bring everyone's mood up so high. Digvijaya would walk away from these ovations beaming.

"This is what I love," he said after one particularly successful meal, "seeing people happy taking the Lord's *prasadam*. This is my meditation, my joy—kitchen religion." Years later, I found a similar sentiment in the words of Carmelite monk Nicholas Herman of Lorraine, better known as Brother Lawrence (1611–1691).[1] Lawrence became a monk in Paris at age 55 and worked as a cook, a service that he considered as sacred as prayer. "In the noise and clutter of my kitchen," he said, "while several persons are at the same time calling for different things, I possess God as great tranquility as if I were upon my knees at the Blessed Sacrament." This, of course, gets at the core of true devotion: there are no times or places where we cannot experience the presence of God.

About 15 years into his monastic life Brother Lawrence walked outside one day and saw a tree. The vision of God's handiwork overwhelmed him. He fainted and woke up about five hours later. After his many years of service and prayer, the simple perfection of nature finally penetrated and something he had seen every day of his life became the impetus for a spiritual revelation. *Prasadam* has that same power: it is God's perfection in the form of food; and when prepared, offered, and eaten in awareness of its connection with God, a meal can lead to a profound awakening.

Apart from this experiential dimension, there is a theology that informs vegetarianism in Bhakti-Yoga and this theology helps explain the transformation of raw ingredients into *prasadam*. Yoga texts such as Patanjali's *Yoga Sutras* and its antecedent the Bhagavad Gita maintain that everything in creation is *brahman*, or divine energy. Eleventh-century scholar-devotee Ramanuja described this by calling food and everything else in the material world "the body of God," a concept reinforced by several verses in the Gita:

> I am the source of all material and spiritual worlds. Everything emanates from me. (BG 10.8)

> I enter into all planets, and by my energy they maintain their orbits. I become the moon and supply the juice of life to all vegetables. (BG 15.13)

> The universe is pervaded by me and by my energies . . . I am the very source of creation. (BG 9.4–5)

> I am the generating seed of all existence. There is no being moving or non-moving that can exist without me. (BG 10.39)

> After many births, those in knowledge devote themselves to me, knowing me to be everything. (BG 7.19)

Yet *brahman* can exist in different states, just as water varies its state from liquid to solid to gas depending on surrounding conditions. Those souls who enter the material world forget their spiritual nature, turn away from the relationship that connects them with creation, and objectify their surroundings. Through that lens of objectified nature, *brahman* assumes a temporary or material appearance. In Bengal there is a saying: a jaundiced person sees everything yellow. Everything that exists may be *brahman*, eternal and unchanging, but in our forgetful state we see the world around us as temporary. Bhakti reforms vision by reawakening awareness of everything around us as nondifferent from God. For an educated Yogi, *brahman* sheds its appearance of temporality and regains its divine nature. Prabhupada offered the analogy of an expert electrician who can employ the same electrical energy to heat or cool. Bhakti scholar William Deadwyler explains that "When 'matter' is used to connect the living being to Krishna [the name for God most prominent in Bhakti culture], then it is acting as internal energy or as spirit."[2] The result can actually be tasted in the offered meal.

"Everyone has tasted these material substances before," says a sixteenth-century Bhakti text. "However, in these ingredients [after being prepared and offered with love to God] there are extraordinary tastes and uncommon fragrances. Just taste them and see the difference in the experience. Apart from the taste, even the fragrance pleases the mind and makes one forget any other sweetness besides its own. Therefore it is to be understood that the spiritual nectar of Krishna's lips has touched these ordinary ingredients and transferred to them all their spiritual qualities."[3]

Compare such an experience with eating in a restaurant or fast-food outlet where profit is the purpose and shortcuts in preparation are the rule!

For those who would cultivate devotion, it is impossible to separate vegetarianism from this shift in vision that Yoga is intended to create. The Christian Eucharist parallels this shift: through prayer, bread and wine transform into the body and blood of Christ. The elements consumed are the same; what changes is the intentionality behind our consumption of them. Sage Patanjali, credited with codifying the codes of Yoga in the second century CE, describes this shift of intentionality as *isvara pranidhana*, or a dedication of all actions to God. Said simply, a nonmeat diet is not in itself spiritual; what renders a nonmeat diet spiritual is devotion. Without the intent of drawing closer to God, vegetarianism qualifies as *sattvic* or materially elevated but not a full-fledged component of Yoga practice. Prabhupada would occasionally remark that pigeons and monkeys are vegetarian, but that hardly qualifies them as great Yogis.

NARCISSISM AND OUR RELATIONSHIP TO FOOD

We have been born so often in so many bodies that we truly believe we are our body and pride ourselves on our physicality. Five thousand years of history since the Gita was spoken have not changed that basic narcissism, and if consuming meat means killing animals so that we can build stamina then so be it. Embarrassing as it may be to admit, on some elemental level we want to survive at all costs, and if I identify myself as my body and its many vulnerabilities then my reptilian brain judges other life as fair game. It is this intractable instinct, not the lack of convincing philosophy, which renders us indifferent to animal slaughter. Relationships don't matter when my survival is at stake. We see this narcissism most vividly in children, who have no hesitation demanding what they want. The raw reality of a child's self-absorption expresses the heart of the human condition: we desperately look for ways to assert our primacy over others because unconsciously we are terrified of dying. We assert dominion because without the illusion of control over our destiny we are left with the reality: we are powerlessness to change it. And that's simply too hard to bear.

My roommate in college was like that. I went to the University of Wisconsin, where many students grew up in hunting families. My roommate was a nice guy, folksy, friendly as can be, but hunting was how he and his brothers had been raised. Eating deer they had killed themselves earned them respect in their father's eyes. During the winter of my sophomore year, he pleaded with me to go hunting with him in the snowy woods near his family's home. We arrived early one December morning, and from the storage room he brought out two sophisticated hunting bows and two quivers of razor-sharp arrows. We walked for about a half hour. Then he positioned me at the entrance to a wooded area while he stalked around back to flush out the deer. Within minutes a stag with a magnificent head of antlers trotted straight across my line of sight. I raised my bow: he was too close to miss. Just as I was about to release the arrow, the bowstring snapped. The bow cracked with a loud explosion. The broken bow flew out of my hands, the arrow shot up into the air and stuck in a branch, and the deer leaped to safety. We drove back to campus in silence. I never had contact with him after that winter, but the image of this unassuming guy playing out his father's fantasy of manhood (and my feeble attempt to keep up) has stayed with me.

Hunting and eating meat have metaphorical meaning for Americans. In the movie *The Matrix*, when Cypher, a Judas-like figure, betrays the Christlike hero Neo, screenwriters Larry and Andy Wachowski place Cypher in a restaurant with agents of the Matrix, doing his deal with the devil while eating a steak dinner and savoring each bite.

"You know," he says chewing with relish, "I know this steak doesn't exist. I know that when I put it in my mouth, the Matrix is telling my brain that it is juicy and delicious. After nine years, you know what I realize?" he asks putting another bit of steak into his mouth and sighing with his eyes closed. "Ignorance is bliss."

Steak epitomizes success. It has had a central role in the mythology of the United States. Meat represents wealth, prosperity, the subjugation of nature, and, despite evidence to the contrary, health and strength. "Meat and potatoes" describes people who are practical, down-to-earth goal-oriented achievers. "A burger and fries" suggests an honest working-class life, real people dealing with real issues and doing their best to feed their children on a modest budget. The food industry has worked hard and spent much to build that image so Americans will continue their habit of consuming meat. And all the arguments in the world won't change someone for whom habit has become embedded in self-image. Many of my students at Hofstra University smoke and drink. They know such habits can kill them, but they still do it. Smoking and drinking are part of a naïve and dangerous campus identity, and the habits won't change until they consider themselves as something more.

CONCLUSION: BHAKTI-YOGA

Bhakti-Yoga poses a challenge to meat consumption not only because it provides convincing arguments about the dangers of meat, karmic and otherwise, but because it offers something more meaningful than the self-image promoted by aggression. When we peel away the awkward illusion of being rugged individualists, we come to the most liberating question of all: how empirically necessary is aggression? Biological history would have us believe it is very necessary, and we have only to consult any of the hard sciences for supportive data. If we insist on biological history as a starting-point for identity, then there is little hope of ever reversing slaughter of any kind. Endangered species acts, human rights conventions and other safeguards will do little to reform behavior that is built into our genetic makeup. Cunning minds will always find ways to destroy life.

Fortunately, the essence of life exists outside biological history. Lasting self-esteem does not depend on aggressive assertion of wants because the core self—the *atma*—has no wants, no identity crisis to resolve and nothing to prove to the world. Uncovering this transcendent self is the purpose of all Yoga, which advocates not vegetarianism but devotion. In stark contrast with the clichéd image of Yogis renouncing the world of the senses, Bhakti-Yogis celebrate the senses as fully part of life's inherent divinity and vegetarian food plays a delightful part in that celebration: as Digvijaya would put it, "kitchen religion." In a world doing its best to counter the consequences of a violent and cruel history, his style of culinary diplomacy may be a tactic worth considering.

NOTES

1. Author Evelyn Underhill offers background on the life of Brother Lawrence in her classic work *Mysticism: The Nature and Development of Spiritual Consciousness*, originally published in 1911.

2. *Gods of Flesh, Gods of Stone*, Joanne Punzo Waghorne and Norman Cutler eds. (New York: Columbia University Press, 1985), p. 82.

3. Krsnadas Kaviraj Goswami, *Caitanya-caritamrita* (Los Angeles: BBT International), *Antya-lila* 16.108–112.

10

❧

Krishna-Yoga and the Spiritualization of Vegetarianism[1]

Steven J. Rosen

Traditionally, there is no Krishna-Yoga. That is to say, the practice of Bhakti-Yoga—the Yoga of devotion to Krishna—has never been called Krishna-Yoga, at least not officially. And yet, if Yoga is linking with God, and Krishna is the primary name for God in the Vaishnava tradition, then Krishna-Yoga is an apt term with deep meaning.

Whatever one chooses to call it, we are talking about a form of practice that has antecedents in the ancient Vedic literature and that can be traced throughout history, as depicted in the Puranas and in the great Epics of India. It was subsequently embraced by the renowned poet-saints and reached perfection in India's major lineage-holders (acharyas), culminating in the life and work of Chaitanya Mahaprabhu (1486–1533). Mahaprabhu's brand of Krishna-*bhakti* was then brought West by His Divine Grace A. C. Bhaktivedanta Swami Prabhupada (1896–1977), and through him, primarily, the world learned of Krishna-Yoga and its uniquely spiritual approach to vegetarianism.

Prabhupada founded his Western Yoga movement in 1965, following in a long line of Krishna devotion and scholarship in India. He called his movement the International Society for Krishna Consciousness (ISKCON), though it is more commonly known as Hare Krishna. Considering our present context, its teachings tell us that if the way to a person's heart is indeed through the stomach, then access to the soul might be found in dietary practices as well. Known for *kirtan* (sacred call-and-response chanting), distinctly Indian dress, and book distribution—at rock concerts, baseball games, airports, and other public venues—ISKCON's message includes the importance of vegetarianism and animal rights in no uncertain terms. In essence, Prabhupada's movement teaches a form of love that is all-encompassing—extending from each member of his society to Krishna and to the entire created world.

Krishna-Yogis see every living being as "part and parcel of Krishna" and thus worthy of their highest affections. Prabhupada elaborated on this point while commenting on a particular Sanskrit verse:

> He [the devotee of Krishna] is merciful because he is the well-wisher of all living entities. He is not only a well-wisher of human society, but a well-wisher of the animal society as well. It is said here, *sarva dehinam*, which indicates all living entities who have accepted material bodies. Not only does the human being have a material body, but other living beings, such as cats and dogs, also have material bodies. The devotee of the Lord is [thus] merciful to everyone—the cats, dogs, trees, etc. He treats all living entities in such a way that they can ultimately get salvation from this material entanglement.[2]

Prabhupada was often quoted as saying, "Real philosophy is nothing more than this: 'friendliness to all living entities.'" Naturally, this sense of universal camaraderie and compassion has far-reaching implications, mandating not only welfare work among humans but also vegetarianism and kindness to animals as well. On a practical level, this manifests in the lives of all ISKCON members as a vow to abstain from eating meat. It also manifests as a plethora of vegetarian food programs, where devotees freely distribute sacred edibles (*prasadam*) to needy people throughout the world. This is called Food for Life (FFL) and has been honored as one of the most important free-food initiatives the world has yet seen, on a par, some say, with the work of Mother Teresa. This same food distribution technique also benefits the rest of society through ISKCON's well-established Sunday Love Feast, where literally hundreds of thousands of plates of delicious vegetarian food are distributed weekly.

Devotees also own and manage many successful vegetarian restaurants around the world, and they are the authors of numerous award-winning cookbooks. In addition, they have established successful farm communities, cow protection (and adoption) programs, and have given the world an elaborate theology of eating—explaining the science of how to determine what is proper food for human consumption and how to turn ordinary vegetarian delights into energizing and sumptuous spiritual fare.[3] Thus, vegetarianism is an integral component of Krishna-Yoga.

The growth of ISKCON in the 1960s coincided with the growth of vegetarianism as an expression of nonviolence in a time of objectionable warfare. That is, ISKCON and vegetarianism enjoyed a contemporary as well as historical synchronicity. In fact, ISKCON in many ways spearheaded the widespread appreciation of vegetarianism and animal rights in the United States and in Europe as well. They did so from the days of their first Sunday Love Feast (in 1966) and continue to do so in the present day. Yet while concern for animals is important in the Krishna-Yoga tradition, its central concern is love of God. This is the real fruit of ISKCON's practice.

THE ORIGINS OF THE KRISHNA-YOGA MOVEMENT

The movement that brings us this precious fruit of India's spiritual heritage was incorporated in New York City in 1966, though it sprouted from the seeds of a religious and cultural system millennia old. These seeds were brought West by Srila Prabhupada, mentioned above, who was instructed to do so by his own spiritual master, Srila Bhaktisiddhanta Saraswati Thakur (1874–1937). Now, an instruction is one thing, and executing it is another. Prabhupada did more than merely take this instruction seriously—he took it to unimaginable places, with a vision and strategic excellence that is the stuff of legend.[4] Colorful ISKCON flowers made themselves visible by the 1970s and continued to blossom into a formidable tree of love of God, offering the world the few fruits mentioned above and so much more.

ISKCON's theological roots can be understood in terms of two historical paradigms, one modern and one ancient. The modern form of the movement reaches back into sixteenth-century Bengal, when Chaitanya Mahaprabhu (1486–1533)[5]—the revered religious ecstatic who fully embodied the movement's teachings, practices, and goals—vibrated a song of universal love. This song's main chorus centered on the chanting of the holy names of God, especially the Maha-mantra, or "the Great Chant for Deliverance": Hare Krishna, Hare Krishna, Krishna Krishna, Hare Hare/Hare Rama, Hare Rama, Rama Rama, Hare Hare, a prayer that means "O Lord! O energy of the Lord (Radha)! Please engage me in Your divine service!"

In the late fifteenth century, European kings sent their heroic explorers in search of new routes to treasure-filled India. Many returned home on ships laden with silks, spices, artwork, and magnificent jewels. But they bypassed India's real treasure, which was just then being widely distributed by Lord Chaitanya. Prior to Chaitanya's time, a reawakening of Krishna-bhakti, or devotion to Krishna, had swept the subcontinent, drawing on centuries-old Sanskrit texts and vernacular poetry composed by Chaitanya's immediate predecessors. Now Chaitanya and his followers were filling in the missing pieces by showing how to put this deep theology into practice and by emphasizing the power of the holy name.

Chaitanya pioneered a great social and spiritual movement that continues to spread its profound influence worldwide. At the very least, he transformed India in four respects: philosophically, by establishing the logic of a personal Absolute named Krishna and the need for rendering loving service to Him; socially, by opposing the blindly rigid caste system and setting in place a universal doctrine that is open to all; politically, by organizing India's first civil disobedience movement against a repressive government; and, most important, spiritually, by teaching and demonstrating that love for Krishna is the secret meaning behind all Vedic texts, the cooling balm to heal all the world's woes, and the ultimate nonsectarian truth for which everyone is searching. It was seen as the perfection of Yoga.

Chaitanya's movement came to be called Gaudiya (Bengali) or Chaitanyaite Vaishnavism, but, as stated, it was deeply rooted in the much older tradition of Krishna-bhakti. To this end, it makes use of standard classical texts, like the *Upanishads*, the *Bhagavad-gita*, and the *Srimad Bhagavatam*. And, in this sense, it is quite orthodox. It claims affiliation with the prestigious Brahma-Madhva Sampradya (lineage), and can trace its teaching to Brahma, the father of the created universe.

This is the second historical paradigm by which ISKCON can be understood. In this context, it is called *Sanatana-dharma*, or "the eternal function of the soul." To briefly elaborate: Chaitanya did not begin his mission to teach something new. Rather, his purpose was to reveal deeper, esoteric truths found at the core of the ancient Vedic tradition. Moreover, his teaching embodies the original spiritual truth found in all religion. Thus, it is not merely Hindu dogma, but, rather, a transcendental science that benefits everyone, regardless of religious or sectarian affiliation.

This, in fact, is what the Hare Krishna movement teaches about its own tradition. Prabhupada faithfully carried on in this same spirit, claiming that his only credit was that he did not change anything, but that he delivered the teaching "as it is." God's revealed word, Prabhupada told his followers, is the Absolute Truth—for our part, we can only follow this Truth and convey it to others, without interpolation or change. Moreover, unlike other gurus and God-men from India, Prabhupada was adamant that a human being should not be identified with God—he claimed of himself merely that he was God's humble servant, and that he was ready, willing, and able to teach others how to serve in this same capacity.

KRISHNA-YOGA: VEGETARIANISM AND ANIMAL RIGHTS

The basic philosophy of Chaitanya's movement is summed up by Bhaktivinode Thakur (1838–1914), father of Prabhupada's guru and one of the premier theologians of the tradition:

Give up the shackles of matter slowly. Cultivate your spirit inwards. . . . Be humble in yourself and learn to respect those who work towards spiritual attainments, no matter what their tradition. Do these with your heart, mind, and strength in the company of spiritual people alone, and you will see Krishna in no time.

Spiritual cultivation is the main object of life. Do everything that helps it and abstain from doing anything which thwarts the cultivation of the spirit. Have a strong faith that Krishna, God, alone protects you and none else. Admit Him as your only guardian. Do everything which you know that Krishna wishes you to do, and never think that you do a thing independently of the holy wish of Krishna. Do all that you do with humility. Always remember that you are a sojourner in this world and you must be prepared for your own home. Do your duties and cultivate bhakti as a means to obtain the great end of life, Krishna priti [love of God]. Employ your body, mind, and spirit in the service of the Deity. Chant His name always. In all your actions, worship your great Lord.[6]

It should be clear from the above that Krishna—famous throughout India as a playful, all-attractive divinity, a dark-hued charmer with a special fondness for cows—is the vision of God in the Chaitanya Vaishnava tradition, and thus the vision adopted by the Krishna-Yoga movement as espoused by Prabhupada. It should also be obvious that abundant humility and its concomitant kindness to all living creatures are central to this Vaishnava path of Yogic religiosity. These factors weigh heavily, as we shall see, in determining the way Hare Krishna Yogis view animals.

A modern-day representative of the Chaitanyaite Vaishnava tradition elaborates on the divine love preached by Chaitanya Mahaprabhu, and emphasizes the positive aspect of *ahimsa*, or harmlessness, which is essential in the philosophy of Krishna consciousness:

Lord Chaitanya propagated the all-embracing philosophy of divine love, irrespective of caste, creed, and religion. Many spiritual paths follow the principle of ahimsa, which means to abstain from doing harm to others. But better than merely renouncing the negative is to be engaged in the positive act of love, which means to do good to others. All animated beings are interconnected and parts of the potency of one all-pervading supersoul, or God. We should realize that our real self is neither our physical body, nor subtle body [mind, intelligence, or sense of identity], but an eternally existing blissful particle of consciousness. Realization of our common relation to the Supreme will foster in us love and affection for each other.[7]

Here we see the fundamental Krishna-Yoga teaching that we are not our bodies but rather that we are spirit-soul, quite apart from the material

body. But, more, we see the basis for true love, that is, that we are all
related spiritual beings with the same universal Father in heaven. The
usual understanding of *ahimsa* is here expressed as a given, implying that
a believing Vaishnava would never cause intentional harm to any living
entity. Interestingly, however, *ahimsa* is now brought further: a *Vaishnava*
is one who feels love for all living entities and performs positive acts of
devotion to help them in any way he or she can. The implications in
relation to our subject should be self-evident.

The movement's specific perspective on vegetarianism and animal
rights is clearly brought out in a conversation between Prabhupada and
Roman Catholic Cardinal Jean Danielou. In a recent academic volume
on the implications of vegetarianism and religion, this conversation is considered in depth:

> The two religious leaders are speculating about why Christians typically
> refuse to extend the Commandment against killing to animals. At one point
> in their conversation, Cardinal Danielou wonders, "But why does a [loving]
> God create some animals who eat other animals?" His answer to his own
> question is both haunting and poignant: "There is a fault in the creation,
> it seems."

> Swami Prabhupada quickly dismisses this possibility. "It is not a fault," he
> insists. "God is very kind. If you want to eat animals, then He'll give you full
> facility. God will give you the body of a tiger in your next life so that you can
> eat flesh very freely. . . . The animal eaters become tigers, wolves, cats, and
> dogs in their next life." The Swami's point is that if there is a "fault in cre-
> ation," it exists nowhere but in the devourer of animal flesh and will be rep-
> rimanded and redeemed in the working out of karmic necessity. Restless
> rapacity is the destiny of the meat eater.[8]

Prabhupada's perspective tells us much about the philosophy of Krishna-
Yoga in relation to vegetarianism, and even something about the nature
of God and the logic of reincarnation as well. First of all, according to Prabhupada, the world behaves according to certain karmic laws, that is, for
every action, there is an equal and opposite reaction. We will explore this
in greater depth later. For now, let us understand that God, by definition,
is perfect and complete, and His creation reflects this same perfection, if
in a distorted way. Prabhupada clearly asserts this faith in God's perfect
nature, and he points out that God is inherently kind as well. The logic
here is simple: if God is perfect and complete, He needs nothing from anyone else, has no envy, and thus has no need to exploit or to be unkind.
Thus, being all-good, He desires our happiness, and He is pleased when
we perform acts that are for our own ultimate benefit.

If, due to conditioning, we desire to eat the flesh of animals—or to engage in any other *tamasic* or violent forms of sense enjoyment, which harm ourselves and others as well—He allows us to do it. In fact, He creates the various species of life—each equipped with a particular sensual forte (e.g., the bear sleeps six months at a time, the pigeon has hundreds of sexual encounters each day)—to facilitate various forms of sense pleasure. As Prabhupada says, "If you want to eat meat, become a tiger." In this way, Prabhupada sees rhyme and reason in creation—the various forms we see around us exist for a reason. More, if we are not at the level of a human pursuing spiritual matters in earnest, we are in effect preparing our next body according to our peculiar desires for sense enjoyment. The goal, Prabhupada informs us, is to learn the true standard of enjoyment—spiritual enjoyment. By engaging in this higher pleasure, he says, our endless repetition of bodily incarnations will end and we can return to Krishna in the spiritual world.

KRISHNA-YOGIS: AESTHETIC ASCETICS

While Krishna-Yoga shares with other forms of Eastern religion a sense of demarcation between spiritual and material worlds—and clearly asserts the living being's identity as a spiritual being encased within a material body—it differs from most other Indic traditions in that its teaching is not otherworldly. Rather, devotees of Krishna exalt in the here and now. True, they shun "sense gratification"—meaning that, as spiritual beings, they prefer not to engage in material pleasures—but they nevertheless enjoy these same senses in a spiritual way. This is based on the precedent set in the *Bhagavad-gita*, where the warrior Arjuna wants to forsake the world and his duties as an administrative officer. Krishna tells him that such weakness of heart does not become him, and that common people depend upon him to do his duty.

Before the time of the *Gita*, Indian philosophy favored the way of renunciation, glorifying the Yogi who goes off to the forest and leaves aside the world for higher goals. The *Gita* teaches something different. It tells us to spiritualize not only our goals but also the actions that lead to these goals. No more should one embrace "renunciation *of* action." Rather, the *Gita* teaches to embrace "renunciation *in* action." The implications here should be clear. We need not shy away from the material world—we need only learn its proper utilization in Krishna's service. This, according to the *Gita*, is true Yoga, or "linking with God."

The virtues of ISKCON's "this-worldly" philosophy have been observed by many, but is most succinctly and articulately conveyed, perhaps, by Steven J. Gelberg, a Harvard scholar and long-time observer of ISKCON:

One can see this spiritual and material utilitarianism in practice in ISKCON in its unabashed willingness to employ the fruits of material technology in spreading its message (vehicles, computers, printing presses, communications technology). It involves not only the use of material objects as such, but also of the body, the senses, and the creative instinct. One can witness this sacralizing of sense activity in the proliferating (and increasingly sophisticated) use among devotees of artistic media such as painting, sculpture, music, dance, and drama to express and communicate the many images, moods, and themes of Krishna Consciousness and Vaishnava culture. This aesthetic dimension is also evident in the construction of lavishly designed temples (such as those in Bombay, Vrindavan, and New Vrindavan), in the use of exquisitely designed dress and ornamentation in the decoration of the temple deities, and in the use of various sensory stimuli such as sound (bells, conch shells, kirtana music), taste (sumptuous food offerings), and aroma (incense, camphor) in the ceremonial worship of the deities. Krishna Consciousness calls not for an extinguishing of senses and sense activity, but rather their purification and elevation through devotional activity. Devotees are esthetic ascetics.[9]

What is being described, then, is a form of inverse Yoga, if you will, wherein divinity is not experienced by suppressing the senses, as in India's many ascetic traditions, but rather by activating them in a unique way. In relation to food, this is clearly a reversal of the traditionally understood need for austerity. It is, rather, a form of "gastro-hyperbolism," wherein the pleasures of the tongue are enhanced, but only in service to Krishna. This focus on sensorial engagement leads to one's becoming a connoisseur (*rasika*), of sorts, developing a certain expertise in determining what is sublime, and what is not.

In other words, through the process of Krishna-Yoga, one develops both esthetic and gustatory "taste"—a word with multiple meanings. In the Sanskritic tradition, its various nuances are found in the words *rasa*, *ruchi*, and *asvada*, all with differing connotations. In short, "the taster tastes the taste with taste." Vaishnavism has thus been called "the kitchen religion," both because its adherents imbibe a distinguished taste for preparing and devouring sacred vegetarian edibles and because it develops in one a taste for Krishna consciousness.

Clearly, this Vaishnava philosophy of spiritual utilitarianism has led devotees into worlds of sights, sounds, tastes, smells, and touch that would be the envy of gross hedonists. It is a realm of synesthesia, where the senses are transformed—heightened—by active engagement in "Krishna Consciousness." Such a transformation is a razor's edge, no doubt, and many a practitioner has slipped, cutting off his or her connection to spiritual life. But those who remain ensconced in the world of the spirit learn of a higher pleasure, one that, again, makes the material variety pale by comparison. As Rupa Goswami, one of Lord Chaitanya's immediate successors and the main systematizer of the Gaudiya Vaishnava tradition, writes in his *Bhakti-rasamrita-sindhu* (1.2.39): "My dear friend, if you are at all attached to the material world, do not look at the smiling face of Govinda [Krishna], as He stands on the bank of the Yamuna at Keshi-ghat. Casting side-long glances, He places His flute to His eager red lips, which seem like newly blossomed twigs. His spiritual body is radiant, and it enhances the beauty of the moon."

If one chooses to look at Krishna's beautiful, smiling face, one cannot simultaneously look into the eyes of a cow that is about to be slaughtered.

THE IMPORTANCE OF *PRASADAM*

The central reason for Hare Krishna vegetarianism is that, according to scripture, Krishna Himself is a vegetarian—and devotees do not eat anything without first offering it to Krishna as a religious sacrifice. In other words, devotees of Krishna naturally prefer to offer Him those foods that He Himself says He would like to eat, and then they accept the remnants as His mercy (*prasadam*). This, say Vaishnava texts, is "the Yoga of eating."

According to the *Bhagavad Gita* (9.27), the entire process of Krishna-Yoga may be summarized as follows, "All that you do, all that you eat, all that you offer and give away, as well as all austerities that you may perform, should be done as an offering unto Me [Krishna]." Thus, offering food to Krishna is an integral part of this Krishna-Yoga tradition. Observing ISKCON and its relationship to food for many years, Eliot Singer writes,

> The act of offering and the prayer which precedes the meal serve to acknowledge that all food is rightfully Krishna's and that the devotees may eat it only due to His "causeless mercy." Offering is a means of expressing subservience. Yet it is also the prime method through which Krishna's "humanity" is revealed. Krishna does eat, although He does not have to do so. In this way, He is explicitly contrasted with the Judeo-Christian God, that "stuffy old man who certainly needs nothing like food." This enables the devotees to feel an accessibility to and intimacy with their God which better allows them to develop the love for Him which is conducive to their concentration.

> Offering *prasadam* is meant to show that man's relationship to God is one of servitude; the devotees receive His leftovers only out of His kindness. Krishna's willingness to accept offerings which are certainly not of divine opulence is also a kindness. This willingness to accept offerings, no matter how humble, is what enables the devotees to develop their personal relationship with God.[10]

In the West, we might wonder why we should offer food to God at all. As mentioned above, He doesn't need our meager offerings—He sustains Himself just fine without them. So what exactly is the point of *prasadam*? Vaishnava tradition tells us that while God does not need our food offerings, as Singer notes, we need the intimacy and deep-rooted connection that comes from offering food to Him. In most religious systems, God is asked for food ("Give us this day our daily bread"), but in Krishna-Yoga, the devotee offers food to God as an expression of love. Even in ordinary dealings, someone might offer us a meal as a sign of warmth and affection. It isn't only the meal itself that is appreciated, but the thoughtfulness and consideration that goes into it. In the same way, the process of offering food to God is intended to help us increase our love and devotion toward Him.

When discussing *prasadam*, Krishna-Yoga texts explain a three-tiered approach to mercy, involving exchange, reciprocity, and redistribution. To make this clear: offering *prasadam* is at the heart of loving exchange with the Lord. It helps us recognize that He initially offers food to us, through the Earth and through mother cow, that is, through nature, and that we can show our appreciation by making a gesture—by offering it back to Him with love and devotion (reciprocity). He then allows us to imbibe the remnants as His special mercy (redistribution).

All religious adherents, East or West, recite prayers over food—and this is certainly an important component in offering *prasadam*—but a closer Western parallel would be the Christian idea of transubstantiation, in which bread and wine are mystically transformed into the body and blood of Christ. The notion of *prasadam* is similar, but it goes much further. *Prasadam* is the essence of the entire spiritual world—it is Radha and Krishna, *and* their loving exchange. It is spirituality in edible form. Moreover, as opposed to the Eucharist, it is not merely a once-a-week wafer—it is every morsel that goes into one's mouth, making it an "all-consuming" act of devotion.

The wafer, it is to be remembered, is not an entire meal, but only an edible symbol. So while the Eurcharist and *prasadam* both represent the reception of God through one's lips, offering spiritual nourishment to all who partake, only *prasadam* actually nourishes the body as well. Thus, *prasadam* is more holistic in that it fully sustains its eaters, whereas the Christian Eucharist is a solitary event, the ingestion of a small wafer and a sip of wine—only once a week or every morning, at best. This distinction is important. *Prasadam* is fully incorporated into the daily life of the Krishna-Yoga practitioner, facilitating an acute awareness of God's mercy, through food and through nature. Eliot Singer remarks on *prasadam*'s all-encompassing symbolism, which reflects the very essence of Vaishnavism.

He perceptively notes how this sacred food resolves the central paradoxes of devotional religion:

> *Prasadam* is a dominant symbol, a symbol which sums up and epitomizes the essential and [apparently] contradictory concepts in Krishna Consciousness: austerity and indulgence, servitude and intimacy, omnipotence and accessibility, suffering and bliss. Prasadam symbolizes simultaneously the austere control of the senses and the celebration of taste in association with the divine. It expresses the duality of Krishna as eater and feeder and of His devotees as givers and receivers.[11]

For those who doubt that *prasadam* is fully spiritual, the devotees remind us that Krishna is supremely powerful. Anything that comes in contact with Him, they say, is overwhelmed by His holy presence. By such contact, even matter becomes completely pure and spiritual, just as He is. Even in the realm of the physical, certain things have the ability to purify various substances. For instance, the sun, with its powerful rays, can distill fresh, pure water from a lake contaminated with pollutants. If a material object like the sun can act in this way, then we can only imagine the purifying potency of the Supreme, who has effortlessly created millions of suns.

Thus, the Krishna-Yoga tradition tells us that Krishna, by His immense transcendental energies, can actually convert matter into spirit, and that He actually does so with offered vegetarian food (*prasadam*). The traditional example is that of placing an iron rod in fire. If one so places an iron rod, before long the rod becomes steaming hot and takes on all the essential qualities of fire, such as heat, smoke, light—it will burn you if you touch it. In the same way, material foodstuffs offered to Krishna become completely spiritualized by lovingly placing them in His presence. This is accomplished by preparing the food with a joyful heart, offering the appropriate prayers, and by devotionally offering back to Krishna the foods He mercifully bestowed upon us to begin with. Food offerings are one of the few commodities that we can share in this way. As one practitioner insightfully says:

> Unfortunately, we can hold onto money, but food cannot be hoarded. It will spoil if it is not shared. A single person can only eat so much food; the rest needs to be shared or it will spoil. Food, then, is the most shareable form of wealth. Food is among the best things that we can offer to God. Whatever we think is best, we offer to Krishna as *bhoga*. Money is not a form of *bhoga*. Krishna is a divine child. If you give him sweets, milk, or other such things, he will be pleased. *Bhoga* is defined as those things that give pleasure to the Lord. Our sect's wealth is concentrated in food. In the Shastras it states that whatever God gives us, we must give back in return, as an offering. Food

should never be prepared for its own sake; to do so is a sin. Why? Because everything we see belongs to God—it cannot be enjoyed by us unless it is first offered to Him. *Prasada* or food is the grace by which Krishna helps us to live our lives. Next to air and water, food is the most essential thing in life. All our necessities, luxuries, everything in short, must first be offered to Krishna, as they rightfully belong to him. We use Krishna's things through his grace.[12]

MILKING THE TRADITION

A related issue, though somewhat tangential, is dairy. While it was never a concern for Krishna-Yogis in previous eras, it is now an important discussion in modern Vaishnava circles. This is because of the state of contemporary slaughterhouses and the mass production of milk. Unlike most vegans, Krishna-Yogis, who base their beliefs on ancient Vaishnava texts, do not think of milk as an unnatural food for humans. The idea is that, in Vedic times, a person lived simply, usually with their own farm and a number of cows.[13] These cows were treated as family, and when they supplied enough milk for their calves, the balance was ingested by the farmer and his immediate kin. This, it was believed, was nature's way, evidenced by the fact that cows usually produced more milk than their calves could consume. It was a lifestyle that was supported by the scriptures and the tradition. Indeed, throughout history, all the great spiritual masters in the Krishna-Yoga tradition were lacto-vegetarians.

But times have changed, with methods of dairy production now as barbarous as those of the meat industry. Dairy cows, let it be known, are tortured in numerous ways. They are forcibly kept pregnant to increase milk production, and shot with numerous chemicals that keep them in a sickened state. They are treated like machines. To add insult to injury, the calves are often separated from their mothers, usually within the first few days of birth. Separation of cow and calf causes untold agony for these creatures, who often bellow out piteously when their offspring are taken away. What's more, male calves are usually killed immediately, at least on dairy farms, since they cannot and never will produce milk—or they are sold to veal farms, where they suffer as their mothers did and are horribly slaughtered. But the dairy cows, too, by 5 years of age, are slaughtered for their meat, even though their natural lifespan could be as much as 25 years. Organic dairy farms are often not much better.

Krishna-Yogis are naturally opposed to these forms of cruelty, for in their tradition the cow is considered all but sacred, dear to Lord Krishna and indispensable for a *sattvic* (mode of goodness) lifestyle. ISKCON founder Srila Prabhupada encouraged his disciples to develop self-sufficient farm communities that could independently supply all their needs, thus circum-venting the horrors of the commercial dairy industry. Regrettably, few such enterprises exist today, though a smattering can be found in Brazil (Gaura Vrindavan), Vrindavan, India (Care for Cows), Mayapur, India (Go Seva project), and in several other parts of the world. As we move into moder-nity, more and more Krishna-Yogis are thus leaning toward veganism if not fully supporting a dairy-free diet.

CONCLUSION

The above might serve as a brief introduction to Krishna-Yoga philoso-phy, a mere "taste" of the Bhakti worldview. It should be remembered that it is through Prabhupada's inspiration and guidance that his disciples man-aged to spread the teachings of Krishna-Yoga, along with its concomitant vegetarianism and animal rights, around the world. As Rynn Berry, author and historical advisor to the North American Vegetarian Society, writes, "Because of men like Prabhupada, the English-speaking world, which was once the most carnivorous tribe on the planet, is now converting to veg-etarianism at a furious pace."[14] And so I wonder: have I conveyed in these pages all that Prabhupada would have me say on vegetarianism and animal rights? Clearly, the *prasadam* factor would be most important to him, and we have dealt with this at some length. An additional but related point would be the limitations of vegetarianism as a spiritual path unto itself. He felt strongly that while vegetarianism is important, people who sud-denly learn of its virtues tend to exaggerate its merit, positioning it, in fact, where God should be. Allow me to flesh this out, if you will.

In recent years there has been quite a bit of talk about animal rights (and its concomitant vegetarianism) as a religious imperative. Animal rights activists with a religious bent say that concern for animals is indica-tive of a superior moral and ethical sensibility. This view is especially held by proponents of the vegetarian movement, which now includes millions in its fold in the United States alone. Some of these "spiritual vegetarians" try to self-righteously shove their dietary preferences down other people's throats, so to speak, claiming that one cannot truly be religious—or be practicing Yoga—if he or she is supporting unnecessary cruelty to harmless creatures. Others quietly practice their culinary spirituality, without preaching to their neighbors. Whatever the case, more and more people see the concern for animal rights as a religious way of life—as a spiritual dynamic that is sufficient in itself.

While this sensitivity to animals is virtuous for the reasons already out-lined in this book, it should not be elevated to a central theological issue, and to do so would be to make it something it is not. The extreme nature of this position becomes increasingly obvious as the ranks of animal rights activists continue to swell. Established religious groups, like the Jewish Vegetarian Society and Christians Concerned for Animals, are well aware of these problems, and while promoting the cause of animal welfare, they are firm in their religious convictions, putting forward compassion for animals as a means rather than an end.

There are others, however, who miss the point, and one wonders whether, for such people, devotion to God (*Ishvara-pranidhana*, as Patanjali phrases it) is being replaced with devotion for animals. True, Jesus said that if one does good "to the least of these, he is then also doing good to Me" (see Matthew 25:34–45). His statement points to an essential "one-ness" between God and His creation, a oneness that all spiritual traditions, including that of Krishna-Yoga, certainly accept.

However, there is simultaneously a great difference between God and His creation, and it is this difference that Yoga traditions tend to emphasize—for only when one acknowledges difference between God and man is there possibility to "unite," to render loving service (*bhakti*), which is the central feature of the theistic enterprise. As one Vaishnava poet sang, "I want to taste sugar; I don't want to be sugar." In other words, it takes two to engage in loving exchange, to feel the "oneness" so characteristic of the Yogic enterprise.

Further, one who places undue emphasis on the creation may thus inad-vertently neglect the Creator. Such illusory misplaced devotion, in which one's allegiance shifts from God to Dog, is becoming more and more common. What one eats is becoming more important than to Whom one prays.

As Prabhupada often said, monkeys and pigeons are also vegetarian, but their spiritual insight may leave a great deal to be desired! Nonetheless, spe-cial interest groups have emerged, and animal rights, like so many other sub-religious concerns, has come to dominate the spiritual sensibility of many practitioners. This is something that deeply concerned Srila Prabhupada.

One can now take a formal Hindu vow of vegetarianism, *sakahara vrata*.[15] The vow may be taken privately, before elders or parents, or as part of a temple ceremony. It reads, in part, "I accept the principle of *sakahara* as the method by which I may acknowledge my compassion, my *karuna*, for all living beings. As an act of dedication, I am resolved this day to begin (or continue) the regular practice of eating a strict vegetarian diet and not eating meat, fish, shellfish, fowl or eggs." While Prabhupada would support such a noble cause, he would be quick to add, "and I will only eat food that is first offered to Krishna with love and devotion."

This, then, might be considered the main contribution of the Krishna-Yoga movement to vegetarianism and animal rights: a truly spiritual dimension. While devotees have offered the world fine vegetarian cuisine, a detailed philosophy of cow protection, free-food programs, a unique take on *ahimsa*, a deep-rooted understanding of universal compassion, elegant and successful restaurants, and some of the most colorful and celebrated cookbooks anyone has ever seen, they offered these things first to Krishna.

I would like to offer one final reflection—a thought that brings me back to my initial attraction to the Krishna-Yoga movement. It is simply this: The *Bhagavad Gita* tells us that the wise person sees all living beings equally, for all creatures are endowed with the spark of life, the soul, and that the outer body is just that—a covering, or an external shell, for the real self. The *Gita* further tells us that God, Krishna, is the supreme father of all who live.

With such an understanding as a basis, we realize that if we deal with God's other children nicely, God will be pleased. But if we try to exploit or commit violence upon one another, how will the supreme father be pleased? And if God's not pleased, how can we expect peace and prosperity in the world?

Animals are also children of God, although they have less-developed intelligence. They resemble human children, or perhaps those with deficient mental capacity (since children may develop into normal adults), who also do not have developed intelligence, or developed speech. Nor can they defend themselves. But in a family, the strong are meant to protect the weak. For a stronger, older brother to torture or massacre a baby is a terrible crime. How upset and angry the father would be! So animals should be treated like our younger brothers or sisters, to be protected, not exploited or slaughtered so we can eat their flesh. "By Krishna consciousness," Prabhupada concludes, "by realizing that God is the supreme father of all living entities, we can actually achieve brotherhood and unity among all living beings."[16] This is Krishna-Yoga.

NOTES

1. Parts of this essay are adapted from my earlier book, *Holy Cow: The Hare Krishna Contribution to Vegetarianism and Animal Rights* (New York: Lantern Books, 2004).

2. See A. C. Bhaktivedanta Swami Prabhupada, trans., *Srimad Bhagavatam*, Cantos 1–9, 30 volumes (Los Angeles, California: Bhaktivedanta Book Trust, 1972–1980), 3.25.51, purport.

3. Cow protection, vegetarianism, and more specifically *prasadam* (sanctified food) are recurring themes in the literature of the Krishna-Yoga movement. An entire volume, *The Higher Taste: A Guide to Gourmet Vegetarian Cooking and a Karma-Free Diet* (Los Angeles, California: Bhaktivedanta Book Trust, 1983),

details the specifics of such sacred vegetarian fare and compassion for animals, as do a plethora of articles in the movement's in-house magazine *Back to Godhead* (BTG). Some of the magazine's more prominent studies on the subject would include Ravindra Svarupa Dasa, "How to Eat in Bhakti-Yoga" (1973); Vishakha Devi Dasi, "Cow Protection: Practical Necessity for a Peaceful Society" (1975); Yogesvara Dasa, "Discovering the Transcendental Taste" (1977); A. C. Bhaktivedanta Swami Prabhupada, "Slaughterhouse Civilization" (published posthumously in 1979); and Rupanuga Dasa, "Diet for a Spiritual Planet" (1980). In addition, for many years the magazine ran a regular column called "Lord Krishna's Cuisine," in which these and similar subjects, as well as numerous recipes, were artfully offered to literally millions of readers.

4. For more on Prabhupada's life and accomplishments from an insider's point of view, see Satsvarupa Dasa Goswami, *Srila Prabhupada-lilamrta*, 6 volumes (Los Angeles, California: Bhaktivedanta Book Trust, 1980–1983). Academic works on Prabhupada and his movement abound. Some of the more important studies are as follows: J. Stillson Judah, *Hare Krishna and the Counterculture* (New York: John Wiley & Sons, 1974); Francine Jeanne Daner, *The American Children of Krsna: A Study of the Hare Krsna Movement* (New York: Holt, Rinehart and Winston, 1976); Steven J. Gelberg, ed., *Hare Krishna, Hare Krishna: Five Distinguished Scholars on the Krishna Movement in the West* (New York: Grove Press, 1983); E. Burke Rocheford, Jr., *Hare Krishna in America* (New Brunswick: Rutgers University Press, 1985); Kim Knott, *My Sweet Lord: The Hare Krishna Movement* (Northamptonshire, Great Britain: The Aquarian Press, 1986); Larry D. Shinn, *The Dark Lord: Cult Images and the Hare Krishnas in America* (Philadelphia: The Westminster Press, 1987); Charles R. Brooks, *The Hare Krishnas in India* (Princeton: Princeton University Press, 1989); David G. Bromley and Larry D. Shinn, eds., *Krishna Consciousness in the West* (Lewisburg: Bucknell University Press, 1989); and *The Journal of Vaishnava Studies*, Volume 6, Number 2, Spring 1998, which was an entire issue on Prabhupada and his movement.

5. For more on Chaitanya Mahaprabhu from an ISKCON perspective, see O. B. L. Kapoor's scholarly volume, *The Philosophy and Religion of Sri Chaitanya* (Delhi: Munshiram Manoharlal Publishers, 1977), and also Prabhupada's own volume, *The Teachings of Lord Chaitanya* (Los Angeles, California: Bhaktivedanta Book Trust, 1974). See also my two volumes, *India's Spiritual Renaissance: The Life and Times of Lord Chaitanya* (New York: FOLK Books, 1988) and *Pancha Tattva: The Five Features of God* (New York: FOLK Books, 1994). For an academic overview of Chaitanya's life and teachings, see my paper, "Who Is Sri Chaitanya?" in Edwin F. Bryant and Maria Ekstrand's edited volume, *The Hare Krishna Movement: The Post Charismatic Fate of a Religious Transplant* (New York: Columbia University Press, 2004).

6. See Pandit Satkari Cattopadyaya, *A Glimpse into the Life of Thakur Bhaktivinode* (Calcutta: Bhaktivinode Memorial Committee, 1916), p. 59.

7. See Swami B. V. Tirtha Maharaja, *The Philosophy of Love: Ancient Wisdom of the Immortal Soul* (San Francisco, California: Mandala Publishing, n.d.), p. 29.

8. See Kerry S. Walters and Lisa Portmess, eds., *Religious Vegetarianism: From Hesiod to the Dalai Lama* (Albany, New York: State University of New York Press, 2001), p. 10.

9. See Steven J. Gelberg, "Exploring an Alternative Reality: Spiritual Life in ISKCON," in David G. Bromley and Larry D. Shinn, eds., *Krishna Consciousness in the West*, op. cit., p. 148.

10. See Eliot A. Singer, "Conversion Through Foodways Enculturation: The Meaning of Eating in an American Hindu Sect," in Linda Keller Brown and Kay Mussell, eds., *Ethnic and Regional Foodways in the United States* (Knoxville, Tennessee: The University of Tennessee Press, 1984), p. 207.

11. Ibid., p. 211.

12. Goswami Krishnajivanji, interview at Jatipura, September 14, 1979. Quoted in Paul M. Toomey, "Krishna's Consuming Passions: Food as Metaphor and Metonym for Emotion at Mount Govardhan," in Owen M. Lynch, ed., *Divine Passions: The Social Construction of Emotion in India* (Berkeley and Los Angeles, California: University of California Press, 1990), p. 169.

13. There were also city dwellings, like Dvaraka, and so on, but the culture itself supported *goshalas* (cowsheds) and a natural lifestyle based on agriculture and a rural economy.

14. Rynn Berry, *Famous Vegetarians and Their Favorite Recipes: Lives and Lore From Buddha to the Beatles* (New York: Pythagorean Publishers, 1993), p. 165.

15. Available online at www.hinduismtoday.com/in-depth_issues/veggie_vow/.

16. This last section is paraphrased from Prabhupada's recorded lectures by Giriraja Swami, "Reverence For All Life," in *Back to Godhead Magazine*, Volume 33, Number 2 (March/April 1999), p. 38.

Afterword

Steven J. Rosen

Though the collection of essays in this book should make it clear that vegetarianism is the ideal diet for the practicing Yogi and that other diets may have deleterious effects on the consciousness (as well as on the body), it should make at least one other point clear as well: Yoga is not about diet.

Without doubt, the point of Yoga is to find union, first in the sense of integrating body, mind, and spirit, and then to link with God, to feel oneness with our Creator. This is easier said than done. Surely, diet can help. A diet in the mode of goodness (*sattva*), as several of these essays have pointed out, is a step in the right direction, and the feeling of compassion for all beings—which naturally manifests as *ahimsa* (nonaggression)—is a necessary byproduct of Yogic practice.

But if moving toward vegetarianism leads to self-righteousness, or a sense of being holier-than-thou, then it is diametrically opposed to the Yogic mindset. In other words, vegetarianism can be schismatic, separating practicing Yogis from the rest of the world, making them feel better than others. Such an inflated conception of self can be as harmful to Yogic practice as eating meat.

What, then, is the aspiring Yogi to do? The answer is actually quite simple. Practice Yoga and try to cultivate goodness in all that you do. This will eventually lead to a harmless diet. Recognize that everyone is on the path and that we all move according to our desire, conditioning, and taste. We are all exactly where we need to be at any given time, and so no one should be judged.

Of course, a teacher's job is to nudge his or her students, to bring them as far as they can go at any given time. And a sincere student will be open to that, even if it is uncomfortable. Thus, depending on how much a given teacher wants their student to reach the ultimate destination, and how quickly, he or she may or may not emphasize a vegetarian diet. Some may even go further, saying that a true Yogi will only eat sanctified food, as in the Bhakti-yoga tradition.

Still, for most, this will occur in stepwise fashion, gradually relinquishing bad habits and eventually realizing the importance of a nonmeat cuisine. In due course, if we engage in the process of Yoga with sincerity and proper intent, we will come to feel love for all creatures, great and small, seeing them as part of God—and, soon enough, we will eat what we need to eat.

In the end, the Yogi should adopt the mood of the Buddha, who said, "And let him cultivate goodwill towards all the world, a boundless (friendly) mind, above and below, and across, unobstructed, without hatred, without enmity." Certainly, such a view will lead to vegetarianism and the perfection of Yoga.

Index

About the Editor and Contributors

Editor

STEVEN J. ROSEN (also known by the Sanskrit name Satyaraja Dasa) is an initiated disciple of His Divine Grace A. C. Bhaktivedanta Swami Prabhupada. He is also founding editor of the *Journal of Vaishnava Studies* and associate editor of *Back to Godhead* magazine. Proficient in Sanskrit, Hindi, and Bengali, he is considered one of America's preeminent authorities on Indic religion and philosophy. He has published more than 29 books, including, for Praeger, *Krishna's Other Song: A New Look at the Uddhava Gita*; *Krishna's Song: A New Look at the Bhagavad Gita*; and *Essential Hinduism*. He is also author of *Gita on the Green: The Mystical Tradition Behind Bagger Vance*; *Holy War: Violence and the Bhagavad Gita*; and *The Yoga of Kirtan: Conversations on the Sacred Art of Chanting*.

Contributors

EDWIN BRYANT received his PhD in Indic languages and cultures from Columbia University. He taught Hinduism at Harvard University for three years, and is presently the professor of Hinduism at Rutgers University where he teaches Hindu philosophy and religion. The author of six books on India-related subjects, his translation of and commentary on the *Yoga Sutras of Patanjali* is specifically dedicated to contributing to the growing body of literature on yoga by providing insights from the major premodern commentaries on the text with a view to grounding the teachings in their traditional context.

DAVID P. CARTER is a longtime practitioner and teacher of Yoga and is minister of the First Unitarian Universalist Church of Wichita, Kansas, where his mix of Western and Eastern wisdom traditions is received gladly. He was initiated into Maharishi Mahesh Yogi's Transcendental Meditation (TM) technique in 1967. After graduating from Maharishi International University in 1972 as a teacher of TM and the Science of Creative Intelligence, he taught the technique to hundreds in the NY tri-state area. In 1984 he met His Holiness Tamal Krishna Goswami and began extensive training in the United States and India, which culminated in his ordination by Goswami as a Gaudiya Vaishnava priest in 1989. Encouraged by Goswami to complement his Eastern credentials by pursuing Western academic studies, he holds a degree in Philosophy and Religion from Southwestern College, Kansas.

CHRISTOPHER KEY CHAPPLE is the Navin and Pratima Doshi Professor of Indic and Comparative Theology at Loyola Marymount University in Los Angeles. His research interests have focused on the renouncer religious traditions of India: Yoga, Jainism, and Buddhism. He has published several books, including *Karma and Creativity*; *Nonviolence to Animals, Earth, and Self in Asian Traditions*; *Reconciling Yogas*; and *Yoga and the Luminous: Patanjali's Spiritual Path to Freedom*. He has also edited several books on religions and ecology: *Ecological Prospects*; *Hinduism and Ecology*; *Jainism and Ecology*; and *Yoga and Ecology: Dharma for the Earth*. He trained in classical Yoga with Gurani Anjali for more than 12 years at Yoga Anand Ashram in Amityville, New York, and initiated the first of many certificate programs in Yoga Studies at LMU starting in 2002. He has been a vegetarian since 1972.

JOSHUA M. GREENE is adjunct professor of religion at Hofstra and Fordham Universities in New York. He is author of several bestselling books including *Here Comes the Sun: The Spiritual and Musical Journey of George Harrison* and *Gita Wisdom: An Introduction to India's Essential Yoga Text*. His books on Holocaust-related issues include *Witness: Voices from the Holocaust* and *Justice at Dachau: The Trials of an American Prosecutor*. He is also producer of numerous documentary films on journeys to enlightenment that are seen on PBS and Discovery.

E. H. JAROW is Professor of Religious Studies at Vassar College, former chair of the Carolyn Grant '36 Endowment Committee on embodied learning and the mythic imagination, and Mellon Fellow in the Humanities at Columbia University. He is author of *in Search of the Sacred, Tales for the Dying,* and the *Yoga of Work*, as well as numerous articles on Right

Livelihood, Vaishnavism, and Indian myth and classical literature. He is a frequent contributor to the *Journal of Vaishnava Studies*.

KINO MACGREGOR is dedicated to carrying the torch of Ashtanga Yoga throughout the world and sharing the tradition of Ashtanga Yoga with everyone who is inspired to practice. She is one of a select few to receive certification to teach Ashtanga Yoga by its founder Sri K. Pattabhi Jois in Mysore, India, before his passing. Perhaps the youngest woman to hold this title, she has completed the challenging Third Series and part of Fourth Series with her Guruji. Each year Kino travels to more than 30 different cities in 14 different countries leading workshops, retreats, and intensives. She and her husband, Tim Feldmann, are the founders of Miami Life Center, a center for Ashtanga yoga, holistic health, and consciousness in Miami Beach, where they also teach together (www.miami lifecenter.com). The creator of three Ashtanga Yoga DVDs and an Ashtanga Yoga Practice Card, she is currently working on her first book. For her full travel and teaching schedule, visit www.kinoyoga.com.

MARGUERITE REGAN is an English Professor at Newman University in Wichita, Kansas, where she teaches courses in writing, British and World Literatures, and Shakespeare, among others. She received her PhD in English from the University of Arkansas-Fayetteville in 2001. Her research interests include eighteenth-century literature and the cultural poetics/politics of food, particularly the rise of a dietary protest literature in England from the late seventeenth to the early nineteenth century. She has also published and presented articles on the use of food and food imagery in the works of James Joyce. In addition to teaching and research, she is a practitioner of Yoga.

Rev. SANDRA KUMARI DE SACHY has been studying and practicing Yoga since 1980. She became a certified Integral Yoga Hatha instructor in 1981 and has been teaching Hatha Yoga, Yoga philosophy, and meditation for almost 30 years. She has an MA in English Literature, a doctorate in English Education, and has taught English in colleges and universities in the United States and in France. Rev. Kumari has written articles on Yoga philosophy and is the author of *Bound to be Free: The Liberating Power of Prison Yoga*, a book that illustrates how Yoga can be used as an effective rehabilitation method in prisons.

NATALIE J. ULLMANN received her master's degree in Psychology in 1991 from The Graduate Faculty of The New School for Social Research and has been practicing Yoga since 1993. In 2005 she was among the first group to be awarded Advanced Board Certification in the Jivamukti Yoga Method, inspired primarily by the emphasis on nonviolence as a fundamental tenet of Yoga practice. For 10 years she served on the faculty of Jivamukti's flagship New York Center, while supporting her work there with studies in food and consciousness with such luminaries as Paul Pitchford and the Wise Earth School. She currently teaches Yoga and traditional food and healing classes in New Jersey.

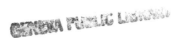